This report contains the collective views of an international group of experts and does not necessarily represent the decisions or the stated policy of the United Nations Environment Programme, the International Labour Organisation, or the World Health Organization.

Environmental Health Criteria 120

HEXACHLOROCYCLOPENTADIENE

Published under the joint sponsorship of
the United Nations Environment Programme,
the International Labour Organisation,
and the World Health Organization

First draft prepared by D.T. Reisman,
US Environmental Protection Agency, Cincinnati, USA

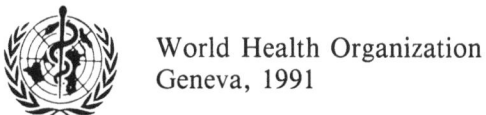

World Health Organization
Geneva, 1991

The **International Programme on Chemical Safety (IPCS)** is a joint venture of the United Nations Environment Programme, the International Labour Organisation, and the World Health Organization. The main objective of the IPCS is to carry out and disseminate evaluations of the effects of chemicals on human health and the quality of the environment. Supporting activities include the development of epidemiological, experimental laboratory, and risk-assessment methods that could produce internationally comparable results, and the development of manpower in the field of toxicology. Other activities carried out by the IPCS include the development of know-how for coping with chemical accidents, coordination of laboratory testing and epidemiological studies, and promotion of research on the mechanisms of the biological action of chemicals.

WHO Library Cataloguing in Publication Data

Hexachlorocyclopentadiene.

(Environmental health criteria ; 120)

1.Hydrocarbons, Chlorinated - adverse effects 2.Hydrocarbons, Chlorinated - toxicity 3.Environmental exposure 4.Environmental pollutants I.Series

ISBN 92 4 157120 9   (NLM Classification: QV 633)
ISSN 0250-863X

©World Health Organization 1991

Publications of the World Health Organization enjoy copyright protection in accordance with the provisions of Protocol 2 of the Universal Copyright Convention. For rights of reproduction or translation of WHO publications, in part or *in toto,* application should be made to the Office of Publications, World Health Organization, Geneva, Switzerland. The World Health Organization welcomes such applications.

The designations employed and the presentation of the material in this publication do not imply the expression of any opinion whatsoever on the part of the Secretariat of the World Health Organization concerning the legal status of any country, territory, city, or area or of its authorities, or concerning the delimitation of its frontiers or boundaries.

The mention of specific companies or of certain manufacturers' products does not imply that they are endorsed or recommended by the World Health Organization in preference to others of a similar nature that are not mentioned. Errors and omissions excepted, the names of proprietary products are distinguished by initial capital letters.

Printed in Finland
DHSS — Vammala — 5000

CONTENTS

ENVIRONMENTAL HEALTH CRITERIA FOR
HEXACHLOROCYCLOPENTADIENE

1. SUMMARY 11

2. IDENTITY, PHYSICAL AND CHEMICAL PROPERTIES,
   ANALYTICAL METHODS 16

   2.1 Identity 16
   2.2 Physical and chemical properties 16
        2.2.1 Physical properties 16
        2.2.2 Chemical properties 18
   2.3 Conversion factors 18
   2.4 Analytical methods 19
        2.4.1 Air 19
        2.4.2 Water 20
        2.4.3 Soil 22
        2.4.4 Biological media 22

3. SOURCES OF HUMAN AND ENVIRONMENTAL
   EXPOSURE 23

   3.1 Natural occurrence 23
   3.2 Man-made sources 23
        3.2.1 Production levels and processes 23
        3.2.2 Uses 24
        3.2.3 Other sources of exposure 24

4. ENVIRONMENTAL TRANSPORT, DISTRIBUTION, AND
   TRANSFORMATION 27

   4.1 Overview 27
   4.2 Transport and distribution between media 29
        4.2.1 Air 29
        4.2.2 Water 30
        4.2.3 Soil 32
   4.3 Biotransformation 35
        4.3.1 Biodegradation 35
        4.3.2 Bioconcentration, bioaccumulation, and
               biomagnification 37
   4.4 Interactions with other physical and chemical
        factors 42

		4.4.1	Phototransformation	42
		4.4.2	Oxidation	44
	4.5	Disposal and fate		44

5. ENVIRONMENTAL LEVELS AND HUMAN EXPOSURE 45

    5.1 Environmental levels 45
        5.1.1 Air 45
        5.1.2 Water 45
        5.1.3 Soil 46
        5.1.4 Food 47
    5.2 General population exposure 47
    5.3 Occupational exposure 48

6. KINETICS AND METABOLISM 52

    6.1 Absorption, retention, distribution, metabolism,
        elimination, and excretion 52
        6.1.1 Oral 52
        6.1.2 Inhalation 56
        6.1.3 Dermal 57
        6.1.4 Comparative studies 58
        6.1.5 *In vitro* studies 60
    6.2 Metabolic transformation 61
    6.3 Reaction with body components 64

7. EFFECTS ON ORGANISMS IN THE ENVIRONMENT 66

    7.1 Microorganisms 66
    7.2 Aquatic organisms 68
        7.2.1 Freshwater aquatic life 68
        7.2.2 Marine and estuarine aquatic life 71
    7.3 Terrestrial organisms and wildlife 72
    7.4 Population and ecosystem effects 72

8. EFFECTS ON EXPERIMENTAL ANIMALS AND *IN VITRO* TEST SYSTEMS 73

    8.1 Acute toxicity studies 73
        8.1.1 Acute oral, inhalation, and dermal
             toxicity 73
        8.1.2 Eye and skin irritation 73
    8.2 Short-term exposure 76
        8.2.1 Oral 76

		8.2.2	Short-term inhalation toxicity	78
		8.2.3	Short-term dermal toxicity	82
	8.3	Long-term exposure		82
		8.3.1	Long-term oral toxicity	82
		8.3.2	Long-term inhalation toxicity	82
		8.3.3	Long-term dermal toxicity	83
		8.3.4	Principal effects and target organs	83
	8.4	Developmental and reproductive toxicity		85
	8.5	Mutagenicity		86
	8.6	Cell transformation		88
	8.7	Carcinogenicity		89

9. EFFECTS ON HUMANS ... 90

   9.1 General population exposure ... 90
   9.2 Occupational exposure ... 90
   9.3 Epidemiological studies ... 95

10. EVALUATION OF HUMAN HEALTH RISKS AND EFFECTS ON THE ENVIRONMENT ... 97

    10.1 Evaluation of human health risks ... 97
    10.2 Evaluation of effects on the environment ... 98

11. CONCLUSIONS AND RECOMMENDATIONS FOR PROTECTION OF HUMAN HEALTH AND THE ENVIRONMENT ... 99

    11.1 Conclusions ... 99
    11.2 Recommendations for protection of human health and the environment ... 99

12. FURTHER RESEARCH ... 100

REFERENCES ... 101

APPENDIX 1 ... 113

RESUME ... 116

RESUMEN ... 122

WHO TASK GROUP ON ENVIRONMENTAL HEALTH CRITERIA FOR HEXACHLOROCYCLOPENTADIENE

Members

Dr K. Abdo, National Institute of Environmental Health Sciences, Division of Toxicology Research and Testing, Research Triangle Park, North Carolina, USA

Professor C. Scott Clark, Department of Environmental Health, University of Cincinnati, Cincinnati, Ohio, USA

Dr S. Dobson, Institute of Terrestrial Ecology, Monks Wood Experimental Station, Abbots Ripton, Huntingdon, United Kingdom

Dr S.K. Kashyap, National Institute of Occupational Health, Indian Council of Medical Research, Meghani Nagar, Ahmedabad, India

Dr F. Matsumura, Department of Environmental Toxicology, University of California, Davis, California, USA

Mr G. Welter, German Federal Environmental Protection Agency, Berlin, Germany

Dr J. Withey, Environmental and Occupational Toxicology Division, Environmental Health Centre, Tunney's Pasture, Ottawa, Ontario, Canada (*Chairman*)

Dr Shou-zheng Xue, Department of Occupational Health, School of Public Health, Shanghai Medical University, Shanghai, China

Secretariat

Dr B.H. Chen, International Programme on Chemical Safety, World Health Organization, Geneva, Switzerland (*Secretary*)

Secretariat (contd.)

Mr D.J. Reisman, Environmental Criteria and Assessment Office, US Environmental Protection Agency, Cincinnati, Ohio, USA (*Rapporteur*)

NOTE TO READERS OF THE CRITERIA DOCUMENTS

Every effort has been made to present information in the criteria monographs as accurately as possible without unduly delaying their publication. In the interest of all users of the environmental health criteria monographs, readers are kindly requested to communicate any errors that may have occurred to the Manager of the International Programme on Chemical Safety, World Health Organization, Geneva, Switzerland, in order that they may be included in corrigenda, which will appear in subsequent volumes.

* * *

A detailed data profile and a legal file can be obtained from the International Register of Potentially Toxic Chemical, Palais des Nations, 1211 Geneva 10, Switzerland (Telephone No. 7988400 or 7985850).

ENVIRONMENTAL HEALTH CRITERIA FOR HEXACHLOROCYCLOPENTADIENE

A WHO Task Group on Environmental Health Criteria for Hexachlorocyclopentadiene met in Cincinnati, USA, from 30 July to 3 August 1990. Dr Chris DeRosa opened the meeting on behalf of the US Environmental Protection Agency in Cincinnati. Dr B.H. Chen of the International Programme on Chemical Safety (IPCS) welcomed the participants on behalf of the Manager, IPCS, and the three cooperating organizations (UNEP/ILO/WHO). The Task Group reviewed and revised the draft criteria monograph and made an evaluation of the risks for human health and the environment from exposure to hexachlorocyclopentadiene.

The first draft of this monograph was prepared by Mr D.J. Reisman of the US Environmental Protection Agency. The second draft was also prepared by Mr Reisman, incorporating comments received following the circulation of the first draft to the IPCS contact points for Environmental Health Criteria Monographs. Dr B.H. Chen and Dr P.G. Jenkins, both members of the IPCS Central Unit, were responsible for the overall scientific content and technical editing, respectively.

Financial support for the meeting was provided by the US Environmental Protection Agency in Cincinnati.

The efforts of all who helped in the preparation and finalization of the document are gratefully acknowledged.

ABBREVIATIONS

ACGIH	American Conference of Government Industrial Hygienists
BAF	bioaccumulation factor
BCF	bioconcentration factor
ECD	electron capture detection
GC	gas chromatography
HEX	hexachlorocyclopentadiene
LAQL	lowest analytically quantifiable level
LOAEL	lowest-observed-adverse-effect level
LOEL	lowest-observed-effect level
MS	mass spectrometry
NOAEL	no-observed-adverse-effect level
NOEL	no-observed-effect level
SD	standard deviation
TWA	time-weighted average

1. SUMMARY

Hexachlorocyclopentadiene (HEX) is a dense pale-yellow or greenish-yellow, non-flammable liquid with a unique pungent odour. It has a relative molecular mass of 272.77 and low solubility in water. HEX is highly reactive and undergoes addition, substitution, and Diels-Alder reactions.

In the USA, the Velsicol Chemical Corporation is the only company that currently produces HEX. In Europe, it is produced by the Shell Chemical Corporation in the Netherlands. Production data are proprietary, but it is estimated that between 3600 and 6800 tonnes of HEX are produced annually in the USA. In 1988, worldwide production was approximately 15 000 tonnes (BUA, 1988). Although HEX is used as an intermediate in the production of many pesticides, some countries have restricted its use in the production of certain organochlorine pesticides. It is also used in the manufacture of flame retardants, resins, and dyes.

During its manufacture and processing, small amounts of HEX are released into the environment. It may also be released when present as an impurity in some of the products for which it is an intermediate. HEX may be released both during and after disposal. Only limited monitoring data on the environmental levels of HEX are available. These data suggest that it is present primarily in the aquatic compartment and is associated with bottom sediments and organic matter except in locations where disposal or release has occurred. In laboratory studies, HEX readily sorbs to most types of soil particles. However, leaching and movement in ground water have been reported.

In the USA, the total annual estimated release of HEX into the environment is 5.9 tonnes (US EPA, 1989). In the Federal Republic of Germany and the Netherlands, about 400-500 kg was emitted to the atmosphere in 1987 (BUA, 1988). Owing to the physical and chemical characteristics of HEX, only a small fraction of these emissions would be expected to persist.

Using the available laboratory data, the fate and transport of HEX in the atmosphere have been modelled and

Summary

a tropospheric residence time of approximately 5 h has been calculated. There have been reports of atmospheric transport of HEX from an area where waste is stored and from wet wells during the treatment of industrial wastes.

In water, HEX may undergo photolysis, hydrolysis, and biodegradation. In shallow water, it has a photolytic half-life of < 1 h. In deeper water where photolysis is precluded, the hydrolytic half-life has been found to range from several days to approximately 3 months, while biodegradation is predicted to occur more slowly. HEX is known to volatilize from surface water, the rate of volatilization being affected by turbulence and by sorption onto sediments.

Owing to its low solubility in water, HEX should be relatively immobile in soil. However, HEX has been found in ground water. Volatilization, which is most likely to occur at the soil surface, is inversely related to the levels of organic matter in the soil. The results of laboratory studies indicate that chemical hydrolysis and microbial metabolism, both aerobic and anaerobic, would be expected to reduce HEX levels in soils.

The biomagnification potential of HEX should theoretically be substantial because of its high lipophilicity (log octanol/water partition coefficient). However, this has not been supported by experimental evidence. Studies in laboratory animals have shown that ^{14}C-HEX is both metabolized and excreted within the first few hours after oral dosing, with little being retained in the body. Steady-state bioconcentration factors in fish are < 30. Bioaccumulation factors derived from short-term model ecosystems indicate a moderate accumulation potential. Therefore, it would appear that HEX and its metabolites do not persist or accumulate to any great extent in biological systems.

Low concentrations of HEX have been shown to be toxic to aquatic life. Lethality in acute exposures (48 to 96 h) has been observed in both freshwater and marine crustaceans and fish at nominal concentrations of 32-180 µg per litre in static exposure systems in which the water was not renewed during the test. Since the photolytic half-life is < 1 h, the HEX concentration would have decreased substantially during the exposure period used in these studies. In the only studies using flowing water and measured HEX concentrations, 96-h LC_{50} values of 7 µg per litre were obtained for the fathead minnow and a marine shrimp. Tests with these two species yielded values for LC_{10} of 3.7 and LC_{40} of 0.7 µg/litre, respectively.

Seven-day static tests with marine algae showed a median reduction of growth (EC_{50}) at nominal concentrations ranging from 3.5-100 µg/litre, depending on the species.

In aqueous media, HEX is toxic to many microorganisms at nominal concentrations of 0.2-10 mg/litre, i.e. levels substantially higher than those needed to kill most aquatic animals or plants. HEX appears to be less toxic to microorganisms in soil than in aquatic media, probably because of adsorption of HEX on the soil matrix.

Although exposure would be expected to be low, there is insufficient information currently available to determine the effects of HEX exposure on terrestrial vegetation or wildlife.

The absorption of unchanged HEX is minimized by its reactivity with body membranes and tissues and especially with the contents of the gastrointestinal tract. Most radiolabelled ^{14}C-HEX is retained by the kidneys, liver, trachea, and lungs of animals after oral, dermal, or inhalation dosing. Absorbed HEX is metabolized and rapidly excreted, predominantly in the urine, less in the faeces, and < 1% in expired air. The terminal elimination time is about 30 h, irrespective of the route of administration. After inhalation or intravenous administration, no unchanged HEX is excreted; the faecal and urinary metabolites have been isolated but not identified. The failure to identify metabolites represents a major difficulty in assessing the pharmacokinetics and potential mechanisms of HEX action.

The acute inhalation LC_{50} (over a period of approximately 4 h) is 17.9 mg/m^3 in male rats and 39.1 mg/m^3 in females. Although there are some interspecies differences between guinea-pigs, rabbits, rats, and mice, HEX vapour is highly toxic to all tested species. It appears to be most toxic when administered by inhalation, as compared with oral and dermal administration, and is a severe pri-

Summary

mary irritant. The systemic effects of acute exposure, irrespective of the route of administration, include pathological changes in the lungs, liver, kidneys, and adrenal glands.

Short-term oral dosing of rats (38 mg/kg per day) and mice (75 mg/kg per day) for 91 days produced nephrosis and inflammation and hyperplasia of the forestomach. No overt signs were noted when mice or rats were exposed by inhalation to 2.26 mg/m^3 (0.2 ppm), 6 h/day, 5 days/week, for 14 weeks. At 1.69 mg/m^3 (0.15 ppm) only mild irritation was seen. Inhalation exposure of rats to 5.65 mg/m^3 (0.5 ppm) for 30 weeks caused histopathological changes in the liver, respiratory tract, and kidneys. A short-term inhalation study of HEX in mice and rats for 90 days showed respiratory system effects at 4.52 mg/m^3 (0.4 ppm) or more. HEX has not been shown to be a mutagen in *in vitro* assays, either with or without metabolic activation. It was also inactive in mouse dominant lethal assays. It has not been shown to be a teratogen in rats and mice by oral exposure; there are no data for the teratogenicity of HEX after inhalation exposure.

Only limited data are available on the human health effects of HEX exposure. There have been isolated incidents in which HEX caused severe irritation in the eyes, nose, throat, and lungs. The irritation was usually of short duration, with recovery beginning after exposure ceased. There were no statistically significant differences in certain liver enzymes between exposed and control groups after short-term exposure. The long-term human health effects of continuous low-level exposure and/or intermittent acute exposure are not known. Handlers of the product and its waste, as well as sewage workers and residents near disposal sites, have been shown to be at risk because of the potential for exposure to the chemical or wastes from its manufacture.

The data base is not extensive or adequate to assess the carcinogenicity of HEX. The US National Toxicology Program (NTP) has conducted a lifetime animal inhalation bioassay using both rats and mice. After the pathology report has been produced, there will be a better understanding of the long-term effects of HEX exposure. An assessment of carcinogenicity will have to be deferred until the results of the NTP bioassay are available. The International Agency for Research on Cancer evaluated the existing data for HEX and classified it in Group 3 (which indicates that because of major qualitative or quantitative limitations, the studies cannot be interpreted as showing either the presence or absence of a carcinogenic effect). Several epidemiological studies were cited in the literature; there were no reports of an increase, attributable to HEX or its metabolites, in the incidence of neoplasms at any site.

2. IDENTITY, PHYSICAL AND CHEMICAL PROPERTIES, ANALYTICAL METHODS

2.1 Identity

Hexachlorocyclopentadiene (HEX) is the most commonly used name for the compound that is designated 1,2,3,4,5,5′-hexachloro-1,3-cyclopentadiene by the International Union of Pure and Applied Chemistry (IUPAC).

Chemical formula: C_5Cl_6

Chemical structure:

CAS and IUPAC name:	1,2,3,4,5,5′-hexachloro-1,3-cyclopentadiene
Synonyms and common trade names:	Hexachlorocyclopentadiene, perchlorocyclopentadiene, hexachloro-1,3-cyclopentadiene, HEX, HCPD, HCCP, HCCPD, C-56, HRS 1655, Graphlox
CAS registry number:	77-47-4
RTECS number:	GY 1225000
CIS accession number:	7800117
EINECS number:	2010293

2.2 Physical and chemical properties

2.2.1 Physical properties

Hexachlorocyclopentadiene (98% pure) is a dense liquid with low solubility in water (Table 1). It is

Table 1. Physical and chemical properties of hexachlorocyclopentadiene

Property	Value/description	Reference
Relative molecular mass	272.77	Stevens (1979)
Physical state (25 °C)	pale yellow liquid	Hawley (1977)
Odour	pungent	Hawley (1977)
Electronic absorption maximum (in 50% acetonitrile-water)	322 nm (log e = 3.18)	Wolfe et al. (1982)
Solubility (22 °C) Water (mg/litre)	1.03-1.25	Chou & Griffin (1983)
Organic solvents	miscible (hexane)	Bell et al. (1978)
Vapour density (air = 1)	9.42	Verschueren (1977)
Vapour pressure (25 °C) (25 °C) (62 °C)	10.7 Pa (0.08 mmHg) 10.7 Pa (0.08 mmHg) 131 Pa (0.98 mmHg)	Irish (1963) Wolfe et al. (1982) Stevens (1979)
Relative density	1.717 (15 °C) 1.710 (20 °C) 1.702 (25 °C)	Hawley (1977) Stevens (1979) Weast & Astle (1980)
Melting point (°C)	-9.6 -11.34	Hawley (1977) Stevens (1979)
Boiling point (°C)	239 at 103 kPa (753 mmHg) 234	Hawley (1977); Stevens (1979) Irish (1963)
Octanol/water partition coefficient (log P_{ow}) (measured):	5.04 ± 0.04 (at 28 °C)[a]	Wolfe et al. (1982)
(estimated):	5.51	Wolfe et al. (1982)
(measured):	5.51[b]	Veith et al. (1979)
Octanol/water partition coefficient (P_{ow}) (28 °C)	1.1 (± 0.1) × 10^5	Wolfe et al. (1982)
Latent heat of vaporization	176.6 J/g	Stevens (1979)

[a] Measured by simple partition.
[b] Measured by HPLC.

non-flammable and has a characteristic pungent musty odour. The pure compound is a light lemon-yellow colour, but impure HEX may have a greenish tinge (Stevens, 1979). HEX (and quite possibly other substances) was reported to have created a blue haze in an accident involving the treatment of waste (Kominsky et al., 1980). A list of some physical and chemical properties is presented in Table 1. It appears that the compound is strongly adsorbed to soil colloids. In spite of its low vapour pressure and high boiling point, HEX volatilizes rapidly from water (Atallah et al., 1980). According to the Handbook of Chemistry and Physics (Weast & Astle, 1980), the ultraviolet-visible λ_{max} in heptane is 323 nm with a log molar absorptivity of 3.2. This absorption band extends into the visible spectrum, as shown by the yellow colour of HEX. Facile homopolar carbon-chlorine bond scission might be expected in sunlight or under fluorescent light. The infrared spectrum has characteristic absorptions at 6.2, 8.1, 8.4, 8.8, 12.4, 14.1, and 14.7 μm. The mass spectrum of HEX shows a weak molecular ion (M) at M/e 270, but a very intense M-35 ion, making this latter ion suitable for sensitive specific ion monitoring.

2.2.2 Chemical properties

Hexachlorocyclopentadiene is a highly reactive diene that readily undergoes addition and substitution reactions and also participates in Diels-Alder reactions (Ungnade & McBee, 1958). The products of the Diels-Alder reaction of HEX with a compound containing a non-conjugated double bond are generally 1:1 adducts containing a hexachlorobicyclo(2,2,1)heptene structure; the monoene derived part of the adduct is nearly always in the endoposition, rather than the exoposition (Stevens, 1979).

Two excellent early reviews of the chemistry of HEX were produced by Roberts (1958) and Ungnade & McBee (1958). Look (1974) reviewed the formation of HEX adducts of aromatic compounds and the by-products of the Diels-Alder reaction.

2.3 Conversion factors

1 ppm = 11.3 mg/m^3 1 mg/m^3 = 0.088 ppm

2.4 Analytical methods

2.4.1 Air

The techniques used to collect samples of HEX vapour in air involve the adsorption and concentration of the vapour in liquid-filled impingers or solid sorbent-packed cartridges.

Whitmore et al. (1977) pumped airborne vapours through a miniature glass impinger tube containing hexane or benzene and through a solid sorbent-packed tube (Chromosorb® 102) tube. Sampling efficiency was found to be 97% with hexane and 100% with benzene. The sampling efficiency for the solid sorbent tube was 100%. The sensitivity of the liquid impinger system was found to be < 11.2 µg/m^3 (< 1 ppb) in ambient air.

Kominsky & Wisseman (1978) collected HEX vapour on Chromosorb® 102 (20/40 mesh) sorbent previously cleaned by extraction with 1:1 acetone/methanol solvent to remove interfering compounds. HEX was desorbed with carbon disulfide (68% efficiency) and analysed by gas chromatography-flame ionization detection (Neumeister & Kurimo, 1978).

Dillon (1980) and Boyd et al. (1981) developed and validated sampling and analytical methods for air samples containing HEX. Methods were reliable at levels below the 8-h time-weighted average (TWA) and threshold limit value (TLV) of 0.1 mg/m^3 recommended by the American Conference of Governmental Industrial Hygienists (ACGIH).

The method developed by NIOSH, Physical and Chemical Analytical Method No. 308 (NIOSH, 1979), used adsorption on Porapak® T (80/100 mesh), desorption with hexane (100% for 30 ng HEX on 50-100 mg adsorbent), and then analysis by GC-^{63}Ni electron capture detection (ECD). The solid sorbent was cleaned by soxhlet extraction with 4:1 (v/v) acetone/methanol (4 h) and hexane (4 h) and was dried under vacuum overnight at 50-70 °C to ambient temperature. The pyrex sampling tubes (7 cm long, 6 mm outside diameter, 4 mm inside diameter) contained a 75-mg layer of sorbent in the front and a 25-mg section in the back. Each section was held in place by two silylated glass wool plugs. A 5-mm long airspace was needed between the front and back sections. A battery-operated sampling pump, which drew air at 0.05 and 2.0 litre/min, was used for personal sampling of workers. The lowest analytically quantifiable level was 25 ng HEX/sorbent sample (using 1 ml of hexane-desorbing solvent and a 1-h period of desorption by ultrasonification), and the upper limit was 2500 ng/sorbent sample. The method was validated for air HEX concentrations that were between 13 and 865 $\mu g/m^3$ at 25-28 °C and with a relative humidity of 90% or more.

Gas chromatography has been considered the preferred method for analysing HEX in air, using either flame ionization collection or electron capture detection (Whitmore et al., 1977; Neumeister & Kurimo, 1978; Chopra et al., 1978; NIOSH, 1979). Gas chromatography/mass spectroscopy (GC/MS) is necessary for confirmation (Eichler, 1978).

Gas chromatography with electron capture detection has been reported to be the most sensitive analytical technique for HEX. The chromatographic response was stated to be a linear and reproducible function of HEX concentration over the range from approximately 5 to 142 ng/ml (25-710 pg injected), with a correlation coefficient of 0.9993 for peak height measurement (NIOSH, 1979).

The lowest analytically quantifiable level (LAQL) of HEX in air was found to be 25 ng/sorbent tube. This level represented the smallest amount of HEX that could be determined with a recovery of > 80% and a coefficient of variation of < 10%. The desorption efficiency of 100% was obtained by averaging the levels ranging from near the LAQL of 25 ng to 1000 times the LAQL (NIOSH, 1979).

2.4.2 *Water*

Since HEX is sensitive to light in both organic and aqueous solutions, the water samples, extracts, and standard HEX solutions to be used for laboratory examinations must be protected from light. The rate of degradation depends on the light intensity and wavelength, the half-life of HEX being approximately 7 days when the solution is exposed to ordinary lighting conditions in the laboratory (Benoit & Williams, 1981). Storing the HEX-containing solutions in amber- or red-coloured (low actinic) glassware is recommended for adequate protection (Benoit & Williams, 1981).

XAD-2 resin extraction has been used to concentrate HEX from large volumes of water. Solvent extraction of water has also proved successful. The detection limit used for the organic solvent extraction technique was 50 ng per litre, as opposed to 0.5 ng/litre for the XAD-2 method. When the solvent extraction method was used under subdued lighting conditions in the laboratory, the efficiency of recovery for an artificially loaded water sample was found to be 79-88%. The authors concluded that the XAD-2 resin could not be used to sample accurately quantitative amounts of HEX in water, but it could be used to screen samples qualitatively because of the low detection limit (Benoit & Williams, 1981).

Lichtenberg et al. (1987) developed methods for the sampling and analysis of organic pollutants, including HEX, in water for the US Environmental Protection Agency (US EPA). Their emphasis was on compound-specific methods, such as GC/MS employing packed and capillary columns. For organochlorine pesticides, methylene chlorine in hexane is used for extraction.

Thielen et al. (1987) developed a technique combining microextraction and capillary column gas chromatography and applied it to plant discharge streams for repetitive waste-water discharge permit analyses. Samples were collected in amber bottles and sealed with Teflon-lined caps. Hewlett-Packard 5880 gas chromatographs equipped with flame ionization detectors, electron capture detectors, and 7672A autosamplers were used for analyses. According to the researchers, the overall effect of converting to the microextraction/capillary-column procedure was both cost-and time-saving, and instrumentation needs were cut by half. A statistical comparison was made to determine whether this technique was equivalent to purge-2nd-trap and normal extraction methods. It was found that the differences in precision were not significant above 2 μg/litre. However, the precision and accuracy of the microextraction method was poor for HEX owing to its instability and the fact that it is adsorbed onto surfaces. The final microextraction data yielded an average HEX recovery (for 44 samples) of 99.27% (S.D. 18.94).

2.4.3 Soil

DeLeon et al. (1980a) developed a method for determining volatile and semi-volatile organochlorine compounds in samples taken from the soil and from chemical waste-disposal sites. This method used hexane extraction followed by analysis of the extract with temperature-programmed GC on high-resolution glass capillary columns using ECD. GC/MS was used to confirm the presence of the chlorocarbons. The lowest detection limit was 10 $\mu g/g$.

2.4.4 Biological media

A method to determine levels of HEX in blood and urine has been described by DeLeon et al. (1980b). This method involves isolation of the compound from the blood or urine sample by liquid-liquid extraction, GC analysis with ECD, and confirmation by GC/MS. The best recoveries have been obtained by using a toluene-acetonitrile extraction mixture for blood assays and a petroleum ether extraction for urine assays. In this method, the detection limits of HEX were 50 ng/ml for blood and 10 ng/ml for urine. Studies by the Velsicol Chemical Corporation have shown that up to 30% of the HEX can be lost if the extracts are concentrated to 0.1 ml. Quantitative recovery is possible only for volumes of concentrate larger than 0.5 ml, which limits the sensitivity of the DeLeon method. However, this method may offer a sensitive process for monitoring occupational exposure.

The Velsicol Chemical Corporation (1979) has developed three analytical methods, which have been used for urine, fish fillet, beef liver, beef skeletal muscle, beef adipose tissue, beef kidney, chicken liver, chicken skeletal muscle, and chicken adipose tissue. The respective recoveries were: 80 ± 10% (1-50 ppb), 81 ± 1%, 69 ± 4%, 88 ± 2%, 86 ± 5%, 71 ± 3%, 55 ± 9%, 76 ± 4%, and 85 ± 2%. The limit of detection for HEX was 0.5 ppb.

3. SOURCES OF HUMAN AND ENVIRONMENTAL EXPOSURE

3.1 Natural occurrence

HEX is not found as a natural component in the environment.

3.2 Man-made sources

Low levels of HEX are released into the environment during its manufacture and during the manufacture of products requiring HEX (US EPA, 1980c). It is also found as an impurity and a degradation product in compounds manufactured from HEX (Spehar et al., 1977; Chopra et al., 1978).

3.2.1 Production levels and processes

Since there is only one producer of HEX in the USA and one in Europe (in the Netherlands), production statistics are considered to be confidential business information and are not available to the public. Production estimates for HEX based on the manufacture of chlorinated cyclodiene pesticides in the early 1970s were approximately 22 700 tonnes/year (Lu et al., 1975). After restrictions were established for the use of some pesticides produced from HEX, USA production estimates were lowered to a range of 3600-6800 tonnes/year (US EPA, 1977). In 1988, worldwide production volume was estimated to be approximately 15 000 tonnes (BUA, 1988).

Commercial HEX has various purities depending on the method of synthesis. HEX made by the chlorination of cyclopentadiene by alkaline hypochlorite at 40 °C, followed by fractional distillation, is only 75% pure, and contains many lower chlorinated cyclopentadienes and other contaminants (e.g., hexachlorobenzene and octachlorocyclopentene). Purities above 90% have been obtained by thermal dechlorination of octachlorocyclopentene at 470-480 °C (Stevens, 1979). The current specification for HEX produced by the Velsicol Chemical Corporation at Memphis, Tennessee, USA, which is used internally and sold to other users, has a minimum purity of 97% (Velsicol Chemical Corporation, 1984).

The nature and levels of HEX contaminants vary with the method of production. The major contaminants found in an industrial preparation of HEX (from Velsicol) were octachlorocyclopentene (0.68%), hexachloro-1,3-butadiene (1.11%), tetrachloroethane (0.09%), hexachlorobenzene (0.04%), and pentachlorobenzene (0.02%). Another preparation (from Shell International Petroleum in 1982) contained up to 1.5% of octachlorocyclopentene and approximately 0.2% of hexachloro-1,3-butadiene (BUA, 1988).

3.2.2 Uses

HEX is the key intermediate in the manufacture of some chlorinated cyclodiene pesticides (Fig. 1). These pesticides include heptachlor, chlordane, aldrin, dieldrin, endrin, mirex, pentac, and endosulfan. Another major use of HEX is in the manufacture of flame retardants, such as chlorendic anhydride, and Dechlorane Plus. It has been estimated that the production volume is split equally between fire retardant and pesticide use (BUA, 1988). HEX is also used, to a lesser extent, in the manufacture of resins and dyes (US EPA, 1980b), and was previously used as a general biocide (Cole, 1954).

3.2.3 Other sources of exposure

Human and environmental exposure to HEX has occurred as a result of releases at production and processing facilities, during transport to disposal facilities, and at land disposal sites.

In 1977, a waste transporter released an estimated 5.5 tonnes of HEX and octachlorocyclopentene, a co-contaminant, into the sewers of Louisville, Kentucky, which led to the contamination of several miles of sewer. The waste-water treatment plant was temporarily closed because of excessive exposure of workers to HEX. (Kominsky & Wisseman, 1978; Morse et al., 1978, 1979). Releases from the Memphis production facility have resulted in high concentrations of HEX in waste water from the facility and have led to HEX being present in the inflow to the receiving waste-water treatment plant and in air at the

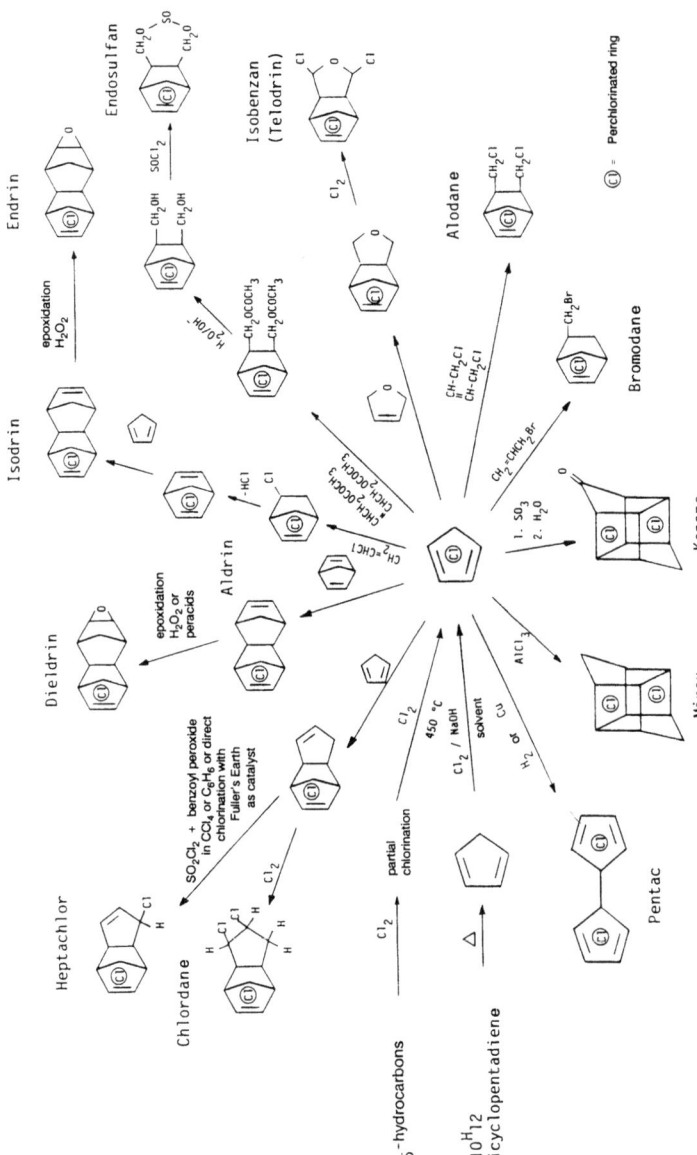

Fig. 1. Synthesis of chlorinated "cyclodiene" pesticides from hexachlorocyclopentadiene (Modified from Bell et al., 1978).

Sources of Human and Environmental Exposure

treatment plant. HEX has also been released from a waste site in Montague, Michigan, USA (US EPA, 1980b).

The US EPA Toxic Chemical Release Inventory for 1987 revealed that over 4.5 tonnes of HEX was released at the Velsicol facility in Marshall, Illinois, USA (most of it from underground injection disposal), that over 540 kg was released at the Velsicol facility in Memphis, and that a similar quantity was released from the Occidental Chemical Corporation at Niagara Falls, New York, USA. The latter two releases were primarily to the air (US EPA, 1989).

4. ENVIRONMENTAL TRANSPORT, DISTRIBUTION, AND TRANSFORMATION

4.1 Overview[a]

The fate and transport of HEX in the atmosphere are not well understood, but the available information suggests that the compound does not persist. Atmospheric transport of HEX from an area of stored waste has been reported (Peters et al., 1981). Experimentally derived constants for HEX in various environmental processes are given in Table 2.

Table 2. Summary of constants used in the exposure analysis modelling system (EXAMS)[a]

Constants	Values used
Water solubility (K_s)	1.8 mg/litre
Henry's law constant (K_H)	2.7×10^{-2} atm m^3/mol
Octanol/water partition coefficient (P_{ow})	1.1×10^5
Photolysis (k_p)	3.9 h^{-1}
Hydrolysis	4.0×10^{-3} h^{-1} [b]
Oxidation (k_{ox})	1×10^{-10} M^{-1} sec^{-1} [c]
Biodegradation (k_B)	1×10^{-5} ml org^{-1} h^{-1} [d]

[a] Adapted from Wolfe et al. (1982).
[b] Extrapolated to 25 °C.
[c] Estimated value (Wolfe et al., 1982).
[d] This is a maximum value based on the observation that there was no detectable difference in the hydrolysis rate in either sterile or non-sterile studies and measured organism numbers (plate counts).

In water, HEX probably dissipates rapidly by means of photolysis, hydrolysis, and biodegradation. In shallow

---

[a] Throughout this chapter, the terms sorb and sorption are used in preference to absorb/adsorb and absorption/adsorption.

water (a few centimetres deep), it has a photolytic half-life of approximately 0.2 h (Butz et al., 1982; Wolfe et al., 1982). Chou et al. (1987) found this first-order reaction to take even less time in full sunlight. In deeper water where photolysis is precluded, hydrolysis and biodegradation should become the key degradative processes when there is little movement in the system. The hydrolytic half-life of HEX ranges from several days to approximately 3 months, and it is not strongly affected by the pH in the environmental range (5-9), by salinity or by the presence of suspended solids (Yu & Atallah, 1977a; Wolfe et al., 1982). HEX is known to volatilize from water (Kilzer et al., 1979; Weber, 1979). It is probable that volatilization is limited by diffusion, i.e. loss from deeper waters should occur very slowly unless vertical mixing has taken place. Sorption on sediments may also retard volatilization.

The fate and transport of HEX in soils are affected by its strong tendency to sorb onto organic matter (Weber, 1979; Kenaga & Goring, 1980; Wolfe et al., 1982). Another possibility is that HEX partitions to the interior of soil particles and stays in loams and silt in a dissolved state. HEX should be relatively immobile in soil because of its high log P value (Briggs, 1973), but several incidents in the USA have shown that this is not true in all soil types (Sprinkle, 1978). Volatilization, which is likely to occur primarily at the soil surface, is inversely related to the organic matter level and water-holding capacity of the soil (Kilzer et al., 1979). Leaching of HEX by ground water can occur, while chemical hydrolysis and microbial metabolism would be expected to reduce levels in the environment. HEX is metabolized by a number of unidentified soil microorganisms (Rieck, 1977b,c; Thuma et al., 1978).

The high lipophilicity and log P_{ow} of HEX indicate a high potential for bioaccumulation. However, in practice, this potential is not realized because of metabolism and elimination. Steady-state bioconcentration factors (BCFs) in fish measured in 30-day flow-through systems were 29 or less (Spehar et al., 1979; Veith et al., 1979). In a model ecosystem study, BCF values for a range of aquatic organisms were between 340 and 1600. These measurements did not distinguish between the parent compound and the metabolites and, therefore, should be regarded as overestimates of bioaccumulation.

4.2 Transport and distribution between media

4.2.1 Air

Little relevant information is available to predict the fate of HEX in the air. Cupitt (1980) estimated its tropospheric residence time to be approximately 5 h, based on estimated rates of reaction with photochemically produced hydroxyl radicals and ozone. The theoretical reaction rates were calculated to be 59×10^{-12} and 8×10^{-18} cm^3 molecule^{-1} sec^{-1}, respectively. In estimating the tropospheric residence time, or the time for a quantity of HEX to be reduced to 1/e (or approximately 37%) of its original value, it was assumed that the rate constants calculated at room temperature for both reactions were valid in the ambient atmosphere, and that the background concentrations of hydroxyl radical and ozone were 10^6 and 10^{12} molecules cm^3, respectively. Direct atmospheric photolysis of HEX was also rated as "probable", since HEX has a chromophore that absorbs light in the solar spectral region, and is known to photolyse in aqueous media. No attempt was made to estimate a rate for atmospheric photolysis. Cupitt (1980) listed the theoretical degradation products as phosgene, diacylchlorides, ketones, and free chlorine radicals, all of which would be likely to react with other elements and compounds.

The vapour pressure and vapour density, water solubility, sorption properties, rapid photolysis (Wolfe et al., 1982), and high reactivity (Callahan et al., 1979) of HEX are significant factors that affect its atmospheric transport. The atmospheric transport of HEX vapour from a closed waste site in Montague, Michigan, USA, was reported by Peters et al. (1981). At an unspecified distance downwind from the site, HEX was detected in the air at concentrations of 0.36-0.59 µg/m^3 (0.032-0.053 ppb). Based on the concentration ratio of HEX and a tracer gas released at a known rate, the average HEX emission rate during the measurement period was calculated to be 0.26 g/h.

4.2.2 Water

In the event of release into shallow or flowing bodies of water, degradative processes such as photolysis, hydrolysis, and biodegradation, as well as transport processes involving volatilization and other physical loss mechanisms, would be expected to play a significant role in dissipating HEX. In deeper, non-flowing bodies of water, hydrolysis and biodegradation may become the predominant processes in determining the fate of HEX.

HEX introduced into bodies of water may be transported in either the undissolved, dissolved, or sorbed forms. In its undissolved form, HEX will tend to sink because of its high relative density, and it may then become concentrated in deeper waters where photolysis and volatilization would be precluded. Some HEX may be dissolved in water (up to approximately 2 mg/litre) and then be dispersed with water flow. The solubility of HEX in water, soil extracts, and sanitary landfill leachates ranges from 1.03 to 1.25 mg per litre (Chou & Griffin, 1983). It tends to sorb onto organic matter and may then be transported with water flow in a suspended form. Transport to the air may occur by volatilization, which has been measured in laboratory studies (Kilzer et al., 1979; Weber, 1979) and was predicted using the EXAMS model by Wolfe et al. (1982). However, suspended solids in surface water may be a major factor in reducing volatilization.

The photodegradation and degradation products of HEX in aqueous solution have been studied in the laboratory (Chou & Griffin, 1983; Chou et al., 1987). When aqueous solutions containing 1.33 μg HEX/ml (a concentration below its solubility in water) were exposed to sunlight, the rate of photodegradation followed a first-order reaction; the photolytical half-lives of HEX in tap water, creek water, and distilled water in sunlight were all less than 4 min. At least eight degradation products were positively or tentatively identified, 2,3,4,4,5-pentachloro-2-cyclopentenone, hexachloro-2-cyclopentenone, and hexachloro-3-cyclopentenone being the primary photodegradation products. Secondary degradation products and other compounds were formed through minor routes of degradation.

A proposed pathway for aqueous degradation is shown in Fig. 2 (Chou & Griffin, 1983).

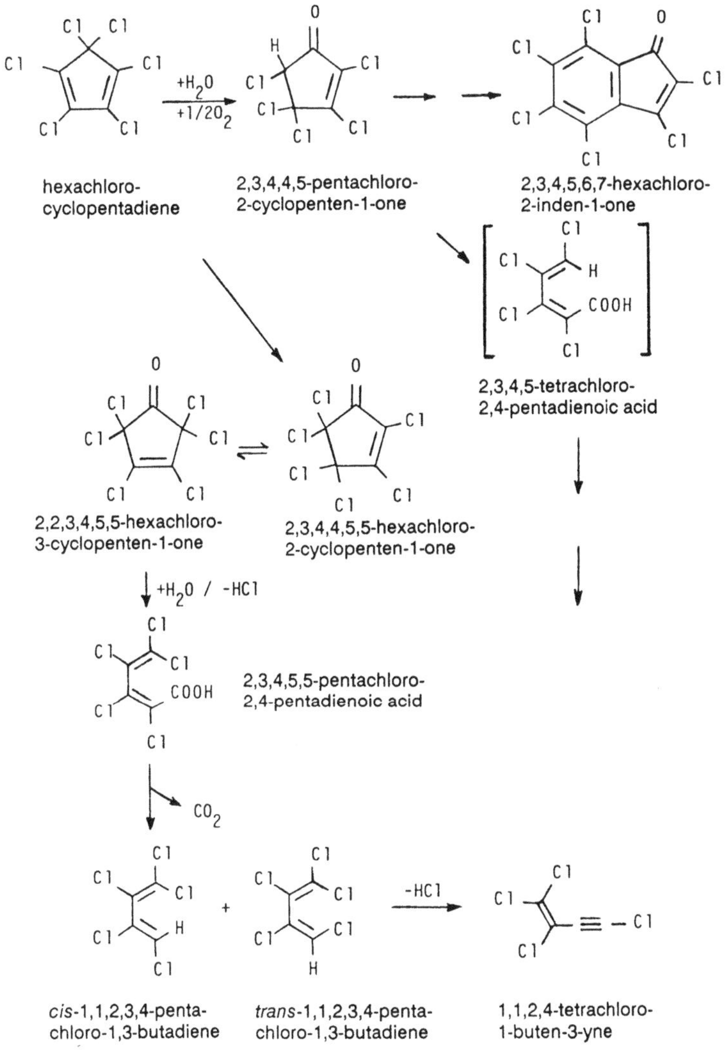

Fig. 2. Proposed pathway for the degradation of HEX in aqueous solution.

Kilzer et al. (1979) determined the rate of ^{14}C-HEX volatilization from water as a function of the rate of water evaporation. Bottles containing aqueous HEX solutions (50 µg/litre) were kept at 25 °C without shaking. The escaping vapour condensed on a "cold finger" and was quantified by liquid scintillation spectroscopy. Based on recovery of added label, the HEX volatilization rates for the first and second hours of testing were calculated to be 5.87 and 0.75%/ml of water, respectively. Since the water evaporation rate was 0.8-1.5 ml/h, the evaporation rates for HEX were within the ranges of 4.7-8.8 and 0.6-1.1%/h, respectively. These results suggest that a fairly rapid initial volatilization occurred at the water surface, and that by the second hour diffusion of HEX to the water surface may have been limiting because of the static conditions of the test. If the rate observed during the second hour had continued for the remaining 24 h, the total loss would have been approximately 18-34%, i.e. somewhat less than that observed in the test conducted by Weber (1979) where unstoppered bottles were shaken.

At 25-30 °C and in the environmental pH range of 5-9, the hydrolytic half-life of HEX was found to be approximately 3-11 days (Yu & Atallah, 1977a; Wolfe et al., 1982). In a later study in which evaporation and photochemical reactions were carefully prevented, the hydrolytic half-life was approximately 3 months (Chou & Griffin, 1983). Hydrolysis is much slower than photolysis (see Table 2) but may be a significant load-reducing process in waters where photolysis and physical transport processes are not important (i.e. in deep, non-flowing waters). Wolfe et al. (1982) found HEX hydrolysis to be independent of pH over the range of 3-10. The rate constant was dependent on temperature at pH 7.0, and the half-life was estimated to be 3.31, 1.71, and 0.64 days at 30, 40, and 50 °C, respectively. The addition of various buffers or sodium chloride (0.5 mol/litre) did not affect the hydrolysis rate constant, suggesting that the rate constant obtained would be applicable to marine environments as well. The addition of natural sediments, sufficient to sorb up to 92% of the compound, caused the rate constant to vary by less than a factor of 2. It was therefore concluded that sorption to sediments would not significantly affect the rate of hydrolysis (Wolfe et al., 1982).

4.2.3 Soil

When it is released on to soil, HEX is likely to sorb strongly to any organic matter or humus present (Weber,

1979; Kenaga & Goring, 1980). The HEX concentrations should decrease with time as populations of soil microorganisms that are better adapted to metabolize HEX increase (Rieck, 1977b,c; Thuma et al., 1978). Volatilization, photolysis, and various chemical processes may also dissipate the compound in certain soil environments.

The main methods of transport for HEX applied to the soil are (a) the movement of particles to which it is sorbed and (b) volatilization. Other possibilities are that HEX is sorbed on to soil colloids or that it partitions to the interior of soil particles and stays in loams and silts in a dissolved state. No data are available pertaining to HEX transport on soil particles. However, in a few studies, the rate of volatilization from soils has been reported and is discussed in the following paragraphs.

Kilzer et al. (1979) found that ^{14}C-HEX and its degradation products volatilized from moist soils (sand, loam, and humus) at a faster rate during the first hour of the study than during the second hour. HEX (50 µg/kg) was placed in bottles with each soil type, the bottles were shaken vigorously, and they were then incubated for 2 h at 25 °C without shaking. The radiolabelled HEX condensed on a "cold finger" and was quantified by liquid scintillation counting. For sand, loam, and humus, the volatilization rate was expressed as the percentages of applied radioactivity per ml of evaporated water. For the first hour the percentages were 0.83, 0.33, and 0.14%, respectively, and for the second hour they were 0.23, 0.11, and 0.05%. For HEX and nine other tested chemicals, the authors found that the volatilization rate from distilled water could not be used to predict the rate from wetted soils. Among the chemicals tested, there was no correlation between water solubility or vapour pressure and volatilization from soils. The volatilization rate for HEX and its metabolites in soil was primarily dependent on soil organic matter content, mainly because of the highly sorptive characteristics of HEX.

In a model ecosystem study, Kloskowski et al. (1981) applied ^{14}C-HEX to 1 kg of humus sand soil (2 mg/kg) and grew summer barley by keeping the system under an illumination of 10 000 lux (12 h light, 12 h dark) at 20-24 °C in an enclosed 10-litre desiccator with an aeration of 10 ml/min. After 7 days, approximately 19.5% of the original radioactivity was recovered in the form of $^{14}CO_2$ evolved and 0.5% as volatilized organics. The level of radiolabelled compounds in the plants was 13.4 mg/kg, which represented a bioaccumulation factor of 7.1 (i.e. plant residues divided by soil residues). It is not clear whether the plants played a major role in the volatilization or metabolic fate of HEX, but the total ^{14}C recovery was over 95%.

Rieck (1977c) measured the rate of volatilization of HEX from Maury silt loam soils. After the application of 100 mg ^{14}C-HEX to soil, the cumulative evaporation of HEX and its non-polar metabolites (penta- and tetrachlorocyclopentadiene) on days 1, 2, 3, 5, 7, and 14 was 9.3, 10.2, 10.6, 10.8, 11.0, and 11.2%, respectively. The results indicated that HEX evaporation to air occurred mainly during the first day after application and was probably associated with the surface soil only.

The soil sorption properties of compounds such as HEX can be predicted from their soil organic carbon/water partition coefficients (K_{oc}). Kenaga (1980) examined the sorption properties of 100 chemicals and concluded that compounds with K_{oc} values > 1000 are tightly bound to soil components and are immobile in soils. Those with values < 100 are sorbed less strongly and are considered to be moderately to highly mobile. Thus, the theoretical K_{oc} value is useful as an indicator of potential soil leachability or binding of the chemical. The K_{oc} values also indicate whether a chemical is likely to enter water by leaching or by being sorbed to eroded soil particles. Since K_{oc} values for HEX are not available in the literature, these values were calculated using the following mathematical equation, developed by Kenaga & Goring (1980) and Kenaga (1980):

$$\log K_{oc} = 3.64 - 0.55 (\log WS)$$

where WS is water solubility (mg/litre), and the 95% confidence limits are ± 1.23 orders of magnitude. The calculated values of K_{oc} for HEX using the reported water solubility values of 2.1 mg/litre (Dal Monte & Yu, 1977), 1.8 mg/litre (Wolfe et al., 1982), and 0.805 mg/litre (Lu et al., 1975) are 2903, 3159, and 4918, respectively.

Since these calculated K_{oc} values are all > 1000, the authors concluded that HEX is tightly bound to soil components and immobile in the soil compartment. Similarly, Briggs (1973) concluded that compounds with a log octanol/water partition coefficient (log P_{ow}) > 3.78 are immobile in soil. Log P_{ow} values for HEX of 5.04 (Wolfe et al., 1982) and 5.51 (Veith et al., 1979) have been measured.

In studies by Chou & Griffin (1983), the mobility of HEX (C-56) in six soils was measured with several leaching solvents using soil thin-layer chromatography (TLC) and column leaching studies. It remained immobile in the soil when leached with water, landfill leachate, or caustic brine, but was highly mobile when leached with organic solvents. A further conclusion was that several degradation products of HEX migrated through soils faster than HEX itself, and that the degradation products warranted further study. The sorption capacity of HEX was highly correlated with the total organic carbon (TOC) content of soil materials (r^2 = 0.97), which was the dominant soil characterization parameter. Sorption appears to be predictable from the TOC content of soils (Chou & Griffin, 1983).

4.3 Biotransformation

4.3.1 Biodegradation

The metabolism of HEX by soil microorganisms is apparently an important process in its environmental degradation. Soil degradation is rapid under non-sterile aerobic and anaerobic conditions, and indirect evidence for microbial involvement has been reported by Rieck (1977b,c). In one of his studies, Rieck (1977b) used several types of treatments and soils of different pH to determine whether the biodegradation of HEX in Maury silt loam soil was biologically or chemically mediated, or both. Soils were incubated in glass flasks covered with perforated aluminum foil and kept on a laboratory shelf, presumably exposed to ambient lighting through the flask walls. When ^{14}C-HEX was applied to non-sterile soil at 1 mg/kg, only 6.1% was recovered as non-polar material (either HEX or non-polar degradation products) 7 days after treatment, and approximately 71.7% was polar and unextractable material. Adjustment of the pH to 4 or 8 had little effect on these results. By comparison, in autoclaved soil (the control), 36.1% of the applied dose was recovered as non-polar material and only 33.4% was recovered as polar and unextractable material. The degradation of HEX under anaerobic (flooded) conditions occurred at a slightly faster rate than under aerobic conditions. However, no sterile, flooded control was used to determine the effects of hydrolysis, which could have accounted for the observed effect in this treatment. The mean total recovery in all treatments decreased from 67% at 7 days to 55% at 56 days. This decrease was attributed to volatilization of HEX and/or its degradation products.

Volatilization from soil was examined in a further experiment (Rieck, 1977c). In a 14-day study, radiocarbon volatilized from non-sterile, ^{14}C-HEX-treated soil was trapped and assayed. A total of 20.2% of the applied ^{14}C was trapped: 11.2% in hexane and 9.0% in ethanolamine-water. Most of the hexane fraction (9.3% of the applied ^{14}C) was trapped during the first day, and probably represented volatilized HEX. However, the ethanolamine-water fraction, considered to represent evolved carbon dioxide, was released gradually over the 14-day period. In the soil analysis, non-polar (extractable) and polar (extractable and unextractable) material accounted for 3.4 and 40.0% of the dose, respectively, during the 14 days; total recovery was only 63.6% including volatilization. No metabolic products were identified in the two studies by Rieck (1977b,c).

Thuma et al. (1978) studied the feasibility of using selected pure cultures (organisms not identified) to biodegrade spills of hazardous chemicals, including HEX, on soil. They tested 23 organisms and found that from 2-76% of the applied HEX had been removed from the aqueous culture medium within 14 days. Seven of the 23 organisms degraded more than 33% of the HEX within 14 days. Losses of HEX by other means than biodegradation were accounted for by using controls.

Atallah et al. (1980) conducted an aqueous aerobic biodegradability study to determine whether HEX could be degraded to CO_2 and at what rate. The inoculum was a mixed acclimated culture containing secondary municipal waste effluent and several strains of *Pseudomonas putida*. ^{14}C-labelled HEX was the sole source of carbon in the study, with the exception of trace levels of vitamins. Total removal of ^{14}C, primarily as volatile organic compounds, was > 80% during the first day in both uninoculated (45 mg HEX/litre) and inoculated (4.5 and 45 mg HEX/litre) media, although removal was slightly greater in inoculated media. $^{14}CO_2$ was released from both media, indicating that CO_2 was a product of hydrolysis as well as of biodegradation. The rate of conversion to CO_2 was initially higher in the uninoculated media, but after 1 week, became higher in the inoculated media. This study showed clearly that HEX can be biodegraded in aquatic media under laboratory conditions. However, Wolfe et al. (1982) failed to detect any difference between the HEX degradation rates in hydrolysis experiments where non-sterile natural sediments were added to water (10 g/litre) and those where sterile sediment was used. They calculated a relatively low value (1×10^{-5} ml org^{-1} h^{-1}; see Table 2) as a maximum biodegradation rate, and consequently biodegradation was estimated to be a relatively unimportant fate process in the EXAMS model (see Table 3).

These studies indicate that the persistence of HEX in soil is brief, degradation of more than 90% of applied HEX to non-polar products occurring within approximately 7 days. Factors contributing to this loss include abiotic and biotic degradation processes and volatilization, although the relative importance of each is difficult to quantify.

4.3.2 Bioconcentration, bioaccumulation, and biomagnification

Bioaccumulation, sometimes also expressed as biological persistence, is a consequence of the rate of elimination of a compound and the extent of adsorption.

The terminology used in this section conforms to that used by Macek et al. (1979):

- bioconcentration implies that tissue residues result only from simultaneous uptake and elimination from exposure to the ambient environment (e.g., air for terrestrial species or water for aquatic species);

Table 3. Summary of results of computer simulation of the fate and transport of hexachlorocyclopentadiene in four typical aquatic environments[a]

	River	Pond	Eutrophic lake	Oligotrophic lake
Distribution (%)				
Water column	1.22	14	12.97	2.91[b]
Sediment	98.78	86	87.03	97.09
Recovery time[c] (days)	52	81	58	87
Load reduction (%) by processes:				
Hydrolysis	8.04	17.85	8.29	16.50
Oxidation	0.00	0.00	0.00	0.00
Photolysis	18.68	80.39	89.18	82.41
Biodegradation (biolysis)	0.57	0.23	0.30	0.01
Volatilization	0.69	1.33	1.56	1.08
Export[d]	72.02	0.20	0.01	0.00

[a] Adapted from Wolfe et al. (1982), with correction applied.
[b] Value was incorrectly reported as 32.91 in original paper.
[c] The time needed to reduce steady-state concentrations by 97% (five half-lives).
[d] Physical loss from the system by any pathway other than volatilization.

- bioaccumulation considers all exposures (air, water, and food) of an individual organism to be the source of tissue residues;
- biomagnification defines the increase in tissue residues observed at successively higher trophic levels of a food web.

The log octanol/water partition coefficient of HEX has been experimentally determined to be 5.04 (Wolfe et al., 1982) and 5.51 (Veith et al., 1979), which would indicate a substantial potential for bioconcentration, bioaccumulation, and biomagnification. Actual determinations of bioconcentration and bioaccumulation in several aquatic organisms, however, indicate that HEX does not accumulate to any great extent (Lu et al., 1975; Podowski & Khan, 1979, 1984; Spehar et al., 1979; Veith et al., 1979), mainly because it is metabolized rapidly.

Podowski & Khan (1979, 1984) conducted several experiments on the uptake, bioaccumulation, and elimination of ^{14}C-HEX in goldfish *(Carassius auratus)* and concluded that this species rapidly eliminates absorbed HEX. In one experiment, fish were transferred daily into fresh solutions of ^{14}C-HEX for 16 days. This transfer of three fish/jar resulted in an accumulative exposure of 240 µg of HEX. Nominal HEX concentrations of 10 µg/litre resulted in measured water concentrations (based on radioactivity) in the range of 3.4-4.8 µg/litre, because of rapid volatilization of the compound. Radioactivity accumulated rapidly in fish tissue, reaching a maximum on day 8 corresponding to approximately 6 mg HEX/kg. Since an undetermined amount of the radioactivity was present as metabolites, no bioconcentration factor could be calculated. From day 8 to day 16, tissue levels declined in spite of the daily renewal of exposure solutions, indicating that excretion of HEX and/or its metabolites was occurring more rapidly than uptake. In a static exposure to an initial measured HEX concentration of 5 µg per litre, uptake of the radiolabel by the fish was to a level corresponding to 1.6 mg HEX/kg on day 2, accompanied by a slight decrease of HEX in the water. By day 4, approximately 50% of the radiolabel had been excreted, and the radioactivity in the water increased. Over the following 12 days, the radioactivity in both water and fish declined slowly.

Podowski & Khan (1979, 1984) also studied the elimination, metabolism, and tissue distribution of HEX injected intraperitoneally into goldfish and concluded that goldfish eliminate injected HEX both rapidly and linearly (the biological half-life was approximately 9 days). The fish (27-45 g) were injected with 39.6 µg ^{14}C-HEX and analysed 3 days later. Of the 97% of the radiolabelled dose accounted for, approximately 18.9% was eliminated by the fish. Of the residue found in the fish, 47.2% was extractable in organic solvent (little of the radiolabelled material could be identified as HEX, which indicated that extensive biotransformation had occurred), 10.6% consisted of water-soluble metabolites, and 20.3% was unextractable. None of the metabolites were identified. The elimination was biphasic, consisting of a rapid initial phase followed by a slower terminal phase.

In another part of these studies, the residual activity in several fish tissues was assayed 2, 4, 6, and

8 days after an injection of 38.4 µg ^{14}C-HEX per fish. The activity corresponded to 0.2 and 0.3 µg HEX/kg in the spinal cord and gills, respectively, concentrations that remained constant throughout the 8-day period of the study. Residues in the kidneys and bile increased within the same period from 1-3 and 0-32 µg/kg, respectively, indicating elimination by these routes. The authors stated that the increase probably occurred from enhanced conversion of the parent compound into polar products, which could be excreted more easily. In the other tissues, all residual levels decreased, leaving only the liver with a level of more than 1 µg/kg. The metabolites were not identified (Podowski & Khan, 1979, 1984).

Veith et al. (1979) determined a bioconcentration factor (BCF) for HEX of 29 in the fat-head minnow (*Pimephales promelas*). In a 32-day flow-through study, 30 fish were exposed to HEX at a mean concentration of 20.9 µg/litre. Five fish at a time were killed at 2, 4, 8, 16, 24, and 32 days for residue analysis. The study was conducted using Lake Superior water at 25 °C (pH 7.5, dissolved oxygen > 5.0 mg/litre, and hardness 41.5 mg $CaCO_3$/litre. On the basis of its estimated octanol/water partition coefficient alone (log P_{ow} = 5.51), a BCF of approximately 9600 would have been predicted. However, HEX did not bioconcentrate substantially, and therefore deviated from the log P:log BCF relationship shown for most of the other 29 chemicals tested by these researchers.

Lu et al. (1975) studied the fate of HEX in a model terrestrial-aquatic ecosystem maintained at 26.7 °C with a 12-h photoperiod. The model ecosystem consisted of 50 sorghum (*Sorghum vulgare*) plants (7.62-10.16 cm tall) in the terrestrial portion, while 10 snails (*Physa* sp.), 30 water fleas (*Daphnia magna*), filamentous green algae (*Oedogonium cardiacum*), and a plankton culture were added to the aquatic portion. The sorghum plants were treated topically with 5.0 mg ^{14}C-HEX in acetone to simulate a terrestrial application of 1.1 kg/hectare. Ten early-fifth-instar caterpillar larvae (*Estigmene acrea*) were placed on the plants. The insects consumed most of the treated plant surface within 3-4 days. The faeces, leaf grass, and the larvae themselves contaminated the moist sand, permitting distribution of the radiolabelled metabolites by water throughout the ecosystem. After 26 days, 300 mosquito larvae *(Culex pipiens quinquefasciatus)* were added to the ecosystem, and on day 30 three mosquito fish *(Gambusia affinis)* were added. The experiment was terminated after 33 days, and the various parameters were analysed. The radioactivity was then extracted with diethyl ether from the water and with acetone from the organisms. The results of thin-layer chromatographic analysis of the extracts are presented in Table 4. Data were not reported for *Daphnia magna* or the salt marsh caterpillar. Uptake in this experiment occurred through food as well as water, and therefore is termed bioaccumulation rather than bioconcentration. Lu et al. (1975) used the term ecological magnification to designate the bioaccumulation factor (BAF). The BAF for HEX in fish was 448 (0.1076 mg/kg fish divided by 0.24 µg/litre water) for the 3-day exposure period, indicating a moderate potential for concentration (Kenaga, 1980). The BAFs in algae (< 33-day exposure), snails (< 33-day exposure), and mosquito larvae (7-day exposure) were reported to be 341, 1634, and 929, respectively (Lu et al., 1975).

Table 4. Relative distribution of hexachlorocyclopentadiene (HEX) and its degradation products in a model ecosystem[a]

	^{14}C-HEX equivalents				
	Water (mg/litre)	Algae (mg/kg)	Snail (mg/kg)	Mosquito larva (mg/kg)	Fish (mg/kg)
HEX	0.00024	0.0818	0.3922	0.2230	0.1076
Other extractable compounds	0.00204	0.1632	0.3824	0.2542	0.1542
Total extractable ^{14}C[b]	0.00228	0.2450	0.7746	0.4772	0.2618
Unextractable ^{14}C	0.00750	0.0094	0.0814	0.0104	0.0982
Total ^{14}C[c]	0.00978	0.2544	0.8560	0.4876	0.3600

[a] Source: Lu et al. (1975).
[b] Sum of HEX and other extractable compounds.
[c] Sum of total extractable and unextractable ^{14}C.

Biomagnification, measured as the ratio of HEX residues between trophic levels (e.g., snail/algae or fish/mosquito), was far less substantial than bioconcentration. Based on the HEX tissue residues, the snail/algae ratio was 0.3922/0.0818 = 4.8 and the fish/mosquito ratio was 0.1076/0.2230 = 0.48.

Lu et al. (1975) also studied the metabolism of HEX by the organisms present in the model terrestrial-aquatic ecosystem, but none of the products was identified except for HEX. The authors reported that unmetabolized HEX represented a large percentage of the total extractable ^{14}C, being 33% in algae, 50% in snail, 46% in mosquito, and 41% in fish. The percentage of biodegradation was calculated for each organism (unextractable ^{14}C x 100/total ^{14}C) and found to be 4% for the algae (in < 33 days), 10% for the snails (in < 33 days), 2% for the mosquitoes (in 7 days), and 27% for the fish (in 3 days). However, these values may underestimate the extent of metabolism, since acetone-extractable polar compounds were not considered in the calculations.

The Velsicol Chemical Corporation (1978) conducted fish tissue residue studies in waters located below their facility in Memphis, Tennessee, USA, and reported that HEX was not detected in either catfish or carp, although chlorinated compounds, including octachlorocyclopentadiene (a common co-contaminant), were detected in the fish tissue. This indicated that HEX was not accumulated. The possible source of these other compounds was not discussed. In a joint USA federal and state study of the Mississippi River at locations above, around, and below Memphis, Bennett (1982) reported that HEX was not detected in any of the eight fish sample groups analysed by GC/MS.

4.4 Interactions with other physical and chemical factors

4.4.1 Phototransformation

Zepp et al. (1979) and Wolfe et al. (1982) reported the results of US EPA studies on the rate of HEX phototransformation in water. Under a variety of sunlight conditions, in both distilled and natural waters of 1-4 cm depth, the phototransformation half-life was < 10 min. Chou & Griffin (1983) determined a half-life of < 4 min at 740 j/m^2. The addition of natural sediments to distilled water containing HEX had little effect on the phototransformation rate. These findings indicate that the dominant mechanism of HEX phototransformation is direct absorption of light by the chemical, rather than photosensitization reactions involving other dissolved or suspended materials.

The direct photoreaction of HEX in water was also studied under controlled conditions in the laboratory using a monochromatic light (313 nm) with a mercury lamp source and appropriate filters. Phototransformation rate constants, computed for the study location (Athens, Georgia, USA, 34 °N latitude), agreed with those observed in the sunlight experiments described above. Rate constants were also computed for various times of day at a latitude of 40 °N. The near-surface phototransformation rate constant of HEX at this latitude on cloudless days (averaged over both light and dark periods for 1 year) was 3.9 h^{-1}, which corresponds to a very rapid half-life of 10.7 min (Zepp et al., 1979; Wolfe et al., 1982).

These laboratory researchers suggested that the primary phototransformation product was the hydrated form of tetrachlorocyclopentadienone (C_5Cl_4O, TCPD), although it was not isolated. Several chlorinated photoproducts with a higher relative molecular mass than HEX were detected by GC/MS analysis of the reaction mixture. Photolysis of HEX in methanol gave a product identified as the dimethyl ketal of TCPD (Wolfe et al., 1982). According to Zepp et al. (1979), it is likely that TCPD exists predominantly in its hydrated form in the aquatic environment. The compound was not isolated, supposedly because it rapidly dimerizes or reacts to form products of higher relative molecular mass. Chou et al. (1987) identified 2,3,4,4,5-pentachloro-2-cyclopentenone, hexachloro-2-cyclopentenone, and hexachloro-3-cyclopentenone as the primary photodegradation products, as well as several other primary and secondary ones (Chou & Griffin, 1983; Fig. 2).

Yu & Atallah (1977b) found that, at a concentration of 2.2 mg/litre in water, uniformly labelled ^{14}C-HEX was rapidly converted to water-soluble products upon irradiation with light from a mercury vapour lamp (light energy: 40-48% ultraviolet, 40-43% visible, remainder infrared). In exposures lasting 0.5-5.0 h, 46-53% of the radiolabel was recovered in the form of water-soluble products (compared with 7% at initiation), whereas the amount recovered by organic (petroleum ether) extraction decreased with increasing exposure duration from 25% to 6% (compared with 66% at initiation). HEX was not detected among the photoproducts in the organic extraction. Chou et al. (1987) also found that dimerization of degradation products to form compounds of higher relative molecular mass was only a minor route of degradation.

4.4.2 Oxidation

HEX would not be expected to be oxidized under ordinary environmental conditions. In the laboratory, HEX reacts with molecular oxygen at 95-105 °C to form a mixture of hexachlorocyclopentenones (Molotsky & Ballweber, 1957). However, based on an estimated second-order oxidation rate constant of 1×10^{-10} M^{-1} sec^{-1} at 25 °C in water (Table 2), the EXAMS computer simulation of Wolfe et al. (1982) predicted that HEX would not be oxidized in the simulated river, pond, eutrophic lake or oligotrophic lake (Table 3).

4.5 Disposal and fate

HEX and HEX-contaminated material and wastes are disposed of in secure chemical landfills, by incineration, and by deep well injection (US EPA, 1989). Additionally, there are solid waste regulations in the USA because, under the Resource Conservation and Recovery Act, HEX is designated to be a toxic waste. German regulations are similar to those of the USA, except that there is no deep well injection (BUA, 1988).

Since the photodegradation products of HEX have been identified only recently and because HEX has also been found in areas where waste has not been disposed of for years (US EPA, 1980c), it is difficult to determine its fate in the environment.

5. ENVIRONMENTAL LEVELS AND HUMAN EXPOSURE

5.1 Environmental levels

5.1.1 Air

Releases of HEX into the atmosphere can result from the production, processing, and use of HEX, the disposal of wastes containing HEX, or from products contaminated with HEX (Hunt & Brooks, 1984). Data sent to the US EPA for 1987 regarding emission levels from companies in the USA indicated that 1400 kg of HEX was emitted into the air (US EPA, 1989). In the Federal Republic of Germany and the Netherlands, about 400-500 kg was emitted to the air in 1987 (BUA, 1988)

In September and October 1985, the Velsicol Chemical Corporation determined concentrations of HEX at predetermined locations around its production facilities in Tennessee, USA. The study was designed to measure ambient concentrations in the air during routine manufacturing operations. Of the 25 samples collected, 15 were below the analytical limit of detection, i.e. 0.03 μg (0.1 ppb). The air HEX levels in the other samples ranged between 1 and 10 μg/m^3 (0.1-0.9 ppb) when ambient temperatures were between 4.4 °C and 27.7 °C (Velsicol Chemical Corporation, 1986).

The highest reported concentration of HEX measured in homes in Tennessee was 0.10 μg/m^3, while air levels at the Memphis North treatment plant were as high as 39 μg/m^3 (C.S. Clark et al., 1982; Elia et al., 1983). In an air monitoring study on an abandoned waste site in Michigan, the average HEX emission rate was 0.26 (± 0.05) g/h. In May 1977, HEX was detected at a level of 633 μg per m^3 (56 ppb) in air samples collected from a waste site in Montague, Michigan (US EPA, 1980c).

5.1.2 Water

Benoit & Williams (1981) sampled both untreated water and drinking-water from a water treatment plant in Ottawa, Canada. Using solvent extraction analysis with a detection sensitivity of 50 ng/litre (or the XAD-2 resin extraction method with a detection sensitivity of approximately 0.5 ng/litre), the authors did not detect any HEX in the untreated water, but reported levels ranging from 57-110 ng/litre in the finished drinking-water. These results suggest that HEX was introduced into the drinking-water during the treatment process. However, the researchers did not find the source of the HEX. Meier et al. (1985) found that HEX can be produced through the chlorination of humic acid.

Limited monitoring data from production sites revealed that HEX was present in a spot sample at a level of 18 mg/litre (February 1977) and a range of 0.156-8.24 mg per litre (over the month of January 1977) in the aqueous discharge from the Memphis pesticide plant (US EPA, 1980c). The calculated concentration of HEX in the Mississippi River was 6 µg/litre (Carter, 1977). In the summer of 1977, shortly after these readings, a new waste-water treatment plant began operation (Table 5). Prior to construction of the plant, waste water flowed directly into the Mississippi River or through one of its tributaries (Elia et al., 1983). Voluntary improvements in controlling the discharge from the Memphis plant resulted in reported levels of 0.07 µg HEX/litre in the Mississippi River, near the mouth of Wolf Creek (Velsicol Chemical Corporation, 1978). HEX has also been identified in the soil and river sediments downstream from a USA manufacturing plant, even after pesticide production was discontinued (US EPA, 1980c).

5.1.3 Soil

Ambient monitoring data for the terrestrial environment are not available, but it seems that these concentrations should be much lower than those in the aquatic environment. Deposition of HEX from the atmospheric (and aquatic) compartments into the terrestrial environment is expected to be minimal. Similarly, direct release of HEX into the terrestrial environment (i.e. as an impurity in chlorinated pesticides) should be decreasing because of regulatory controls on some products, with the possible exceptions of disposal at waste sites, accidental spills, and other illegal disposal methods.

Table 5. Concentrations of selected organic compounds in influent waste water at the Memphis North treatment plant, 1978[a]

Date	No. of samples	Concentration (µg/litre)[b]			
		HEX	HEX-BCH[c]	HCBCH[d]	Chlordane
June	1	3	334	57	87
August	5	0.8	329	115	216
September	2	4	292	668	58
October-November	2	0.8	11	17	32

[a] From: Elia et al. (1983).
[b] Mean values for the number of samples indicated.
[c] Hexachlorobicycloheptadiene.
[d] Heptachlorobicycloheptene.

5.1.4 Food

HEX was qualitatively detected in fish samples taken from water near a pesticide manufacturing plant in Michigan (Spehar et al., 1977), but none was detected in fish samples taken from the waters near the pesticide manufacturing plant in Memphis (Velsicol Chemical Corporation, 1978; Bennett, 1982). No information regarding HEX contamination of other foods is available.

5.2 General population exposure

There are insufficient data to determine the relative contributions of the various sources of HEX to the environment. There will be exposure to HEX present in some commonly used pesticides, and possibly some flame retardants, where HEX is a contaminant. The US EPA has reported that exposure of humans to HEX from the air or water should be extremely low, except in the case of workers and residents near manufacturing, shipping, and waste sites, and concluded that general population exposure was not considered to be significant or substantial (US EPA, 1982).

The only other estimates of relative source contributions are from reports completed for the US EPA (Hunt & Brooks, 1984) and the BUA (1988). The air releases from manufacturing processes can come from the vents on reactors, process and storage tanks, and as fugitive emissions. Hunt & Brooks (1984) estimated that the total quantity of HEX released from these sources was 8 tonnes per year. In the Federal Republic of Germany and the Netherlands, HEX emissions were estimated to be 400-500 kg/year. HEX can also be emitted into the air from the incineration and landfilling of HEX-containing waste, the most accurate estimate being 1 tonne per year. The total annual estimated release of HEX to the environment in the USA is 11.9 tonnes. These figures are only estimates because of the limited available data. They are given simply to indicate the relative magnitude of HEX emissions into the environment.

Exposure limit values for various countries are given in Appendix 1.

5.3 Occupational exposure

Occupational exposure can occur both at HEX production and processing facilities and at other locations where HEX-containing waste is present. For example, the highest reported workplace air concentrations of HEX were measured at the Louisville, Kentucky, USA, waste-water treatment plant, which received a slug of HEX discharged by a waste hauler. Four days after the plant was closed, air concentrations in the primary treatment area ranged from 3.05 to 11.0 mg/m^3 (270 to 970 ppb) (Morse et al., 1979). During the clean-up operations air concentrations as high as 133 mg/m^3 (11 800 ppb) were reported (Kominsky & Wisseman, 1978).

In 1982, the Velsicol Chemical Corporation used the Southern Research Institute (SRI) sampling method at the Memphis (Tennessee) and Marshall (Illinois) facilities to evaluate possible exposure of workers to HEX vapour and the effectiveness of engineering controls. Tables 6 and 7 show the HEX concentrations measured at various points.

At the Memphis facility almost one-half of the worker 8-h time-weighted average (TWA) air HEX concentrations were at or above the USA Threshold Limit Value of 0.11 mg/m^3 (0.01 ppm) (OSHA, 1989). At the Marshall plant all six TWA values were above 0.11 mg/m^3. It should be noted that in Tables 6 and 7 the results of employee monitoring are reported without regard to respirator use. Respirators are required to be worn in operations in these plants where HEX exposure is possible.

Information on guidelines, recommendations, and standards used in various countries is given in Appendix 1 (Table 21).

Table 6. Summary of hexachlorocyclopentadiene monitoring, Memphis, Tennessee, USA[a]

Unit	Description	No. of samples	Average duration (min)	Range of sample concentrations[b] (ppm)	Average TWA[b] (ppm)
HEX	Process operator	2	445	0.009-0.011	0.009
HEX	No. 1 operator	5	432	0.006-0.033	0.015
HEX	No. 2 process operator	5	418	0.006-0.029	0.014
HEX	No. 2 cyclo operator	5	417	0.001-0.048	0.017
HEX	No. 2 chlorine operator	6	415	0.004-0.0161	0.035
	a) HEX Bottoms drumming	1	50	0.016	
HEX	Area sample control room	12	476	0.002-0.018	0.009
HEX	Brinks filter cleaning	2	387	0.004-0.006	0.005
Formulations	HEX drummers	4	407	0.002-2.0337	0.010
Material handling	HEX railroad tank car unloading	1	279	0.013	0.008
Endrin	R2 filter operator	1	281	0.003	
Endrin	R1 operator	1	334	0.002	
Chlorendic anhydride	No. 1 operator	2	437	0.0077-0.0102	0.008
Chlorendic anhydride	No. 2 operator D34	2	440	0.0107-0.0198	0.014
Chlorendic anhydride	No. 2 operator R6	2	437	0.0065-0.0169	0.011
Chlorendic anhydride	Packaging operator	1	396	0.035	0.031
Chlorendic anhydride	Area sample - control room	3	475	0.0003-0.0014	0.001
Heptachlor	No. 1 operator	2	407	0.007-0.009	0.007
Heptachlor	No. 2 operator	2	415	0.006-0.009	0.007
Heptachlor	237 operator	2	392	0.006-0.019	0.011
Heptachlor	Utility operator	1	363	0.006	0.005
Heptachlor	Cleaning sparkler filter	3	44	0.002-0.005	0.0003
	a) ceiling sample	1	15	0.006	

[a] From: Levin (1982a).
[b] ppm = parts of HEX per million parts of air by volume.
TWA = 8-h time-weighted average. The TWA calculation was made assuming that the only chemical exposure occurred during the sampling period.

Table 7. Summary of hexachlorocyclopentadiene monitoring, Marshall, Illinois, USA[a]

Unit	Description	No. of samples	Average duration (min)	Range of sample concentrations (ppm)	Average TWA[b] (ppm)
Chlordane	No. 1 operator	8	451	0.0091-0.0316	0.017
Chlordane	No. 2 operator	8	455	0.008-0.0195	0.013
Chlordane	No. 3 operator	8	451	0.0002-0.0325	0.014
Chlordane	Area sample - North control room	13	433	0.0002-0.0254	0.016
Chlordane	Area sample - South control room	10	435	0.001-0.0276	0.015
Chlordane	HEX filter changing	1	15	0.1322	
Chlordane	Waste handling HEX	6	307	0.0006-0.0606	0.020
	a) HEX mud drumming - ceiling sample	2	15	0.0005-0.0061	
	b) Loading HEX waste truck - ceiling sample	2	15	0.1199-0.2325	
	c) Sump pit dumping - ceiling sample	2	15	0.0333-0.1129	

[a] From: Levin (1982a).
[b] ppm = parts of HEX per million parts of air by volume.
TWA = 8-h time-weighted average. The TWA calculation was made assuming that the only chemical exposure was during the sampling period.

6. KINETICS AND METABOLISM

6.1 Absorption, retention, distribution, metabolism, elimination, and excretion

6.1.1 Oral

In a study by Mehendale (1977), male Sprague-Dawley rats (225-250 g body weight) were administered 5 µmol of ^{14}C-HEX (approximately 5.5 mg/kg) by oral intubation as 0.2 ml of a solution in corn oil. The total ^{14}C activity contained in the dose was approximately 1 µCi. The animals were maintained in metabolism cages and the urine and faeces were collected. About 35% of the administered dose was collected in the urine and only 10% was collected in the faeces. More than 87% of the ^{14}C activity in the urine and more than 60% of the activity in the faeces appeared during the first day. Only a small amount (approximately 0.5%) of the original dose was recovered in the kidneys and liver. The author speculated that, in view of the low total recovery of the administered dose, a major part of the dose (> 50%) had been excreted through the lung. This speculation was later proven to be unwarranted because subsequent studies (Dorough, 1979), in which exhaled air and lung and tracheal tissues were analysed, showed that this was not the case. There is strong evidence to suggest that, after oral dosing with HEX, at least part of the faecal contents contained a volatile constituent that could be readily lost if the samples were dried and powdered, as they were in this case. An extraction procedure, using the major tissues and excreta, followed by thin-layer chromatography, showed that at least four water-soluble (polar) metabolites were produced, but not identified, after oral dosing.

In a study designed to re-examine some of the findings and observations of Mehendale (1977), Dorough (1979) investigated the accumulation, distribution, and excretion of ^{14}C-HEX after its administration to rats and mice either as a single oral dose or as a component of their diet. The principal results of this study were reported by Dorough & Ranieri (1984). The animals used were male and female Sprague-Dawley rats, weighing between 200 and 250 g body weight, and male and female Sprague-Dawley albino mice, weighing between 25 and 30 g. Two female rats were dosed, by gavage, with HEX (20 mg/kg) in 0.9 ml of corn oil and were immediately placed in separate metabolism cages through which air was drawn at 600 ml/min. The evacuated air was passed through two high efficiency traps. Since less than 1% of the administered dose was recovered from the traps, it was considered to be conclusive evidence that the pulmonary route is not of major importance in the excretion of HEX (Dorough, 1979).

Dorough (1979) conducted single dose studies by administering, with a dosing needle, either 2.5 or 25 mg ^{14}C-HEX/kg body weight (dissolved in 0.9 ml of corn oil for rats and in 0.2-0.3 ml for mice). The animals were killed at 1, 3, or 7 days after dosing, and samples of muscle, brain, liver, kidneys, fat, and either ovaries or testes were removed and analysed for ^{14}C activity. Urine and faeces were also collected during the period between dosing and tissue sample collection. No appreciable differences due to sex or species were found in the excretion patterns. The liver, kidneys, and fat were the most important deposition sites for ^{14}C residues in both rats and mice, the levels in the kidneys of rats and in the liver of mice being the highest.

In the same study (Dorough, 1979), rats and mice were also placed on diets containing 1, 5, or 25 mg ^{14}C-HEX per kg. Assuming a daily food intake of 15 g for rats and 5 g for mice, this would give daily dose rates of 0.066, 0.330, and 1.666 mg/kg for rats and 0.182, 0.910, and 4.55 mg/kg for mice. Feed was replaced in the feeders every 12 h to minimize the loss of ^{14}C-HEX (from volatilization), and the feeding study was carried out for 30 days. During this period, rats and mice were killed at 1, 3, 7, 12, 15, or 30 days. The surviving animals were then returned to a normal diet for up to 30 days and, during this post-treatment period, animals were killed at 1, 3, 7, 15, or 30 days after the last exposure. The total excretion (urine and faeces) of the radiolabel ranged from 63-79% of the consumed ^{14}C-HEX, which was significantly lower than that found in the single-dose study (73-96%). In all cases, the liver, kidneys, and fat contained the highest amounts of ^{14}C, and it appeared that a steady state for these levels was reached after 15 days of the feeding phase. A good correlation was observed between the level of HEX in the diet and the ^{14}C-levels found in all the examined tissues. In a separate experiment with male rats, in which the bile duct was cannulated and a single dose of ^{14}C-HEX (25 mg/kg) was administered orally, only 16% of the dose was excreted in the bile. The extraction characteristics of the radiocarbon compounds in the excreta showed that they were primarily polar metabolites, some of which were capable of being converted to organic-soluble compounds after acid-catalysed hydrolysis.

In a comparative study of the pharmacokinetics of ^{14}C-HEX after intravenous and oral dosing, Yu & Atallah (1981) dosed Sprague-Dawley rats (240-350 g body weight) with either 3 or 6 mg ^{14}C-HEX (specific activity: 0.267 mCi/mmol). The doses ranged from 8.5 to 25.6 mg/kg. Shortly after oral dosing, ^{14}C activity appeared in the blood and reached a maximum after approximately 4 h.

The ^{14}C activity appeared in most of the tissues analysed at 8, 24, 48, 72, 96, and 120 h after dosing. Following oral dosing, there were higher residue levels in the kidneys and liver than in any other tissue, although these levels were generally much lower than those observed after intravenous dosing. For example, at 24 h after dosing, the kidneys and liver were found to contain only 0.96 and 0.75%, respectively, of the administered oral dose, while these organs retained 2.92 and 4.68%, respectively, of the administered intravenous dose. A higher proportion (15.07%) of the ^{14}C activity was found in the digestive system (duodenum and large and small intestines) after oral dosing. Coupled with the increased rate and extent of faecal excretion after oral administration (approximately 72%), compared to that after intravenous dosing (approximately 20%), this would suggest that only a fraction of the orally administered dose was absorbed. About 17% of the oral dose was excreted in the urine.

Both urinary and faecal metabolites were again characterized as polar because of their insolubility in organic solvents. Unchanged HEX was not detected in any of the samples examined. Only 11% of the ^{14}C content was soluble in organic solvents and a further 32% was converted to organic-soluble compounds after acid-catalysed hydrolysis. This indicated, perhaps, the formation of metabolic ester conjugates.

Lawrence & Dorough (1982) made a comparative study of the uptake, disposition, and elimination of HEX after administering radiolabelled ^{14}C-HEX by the intravenous (10 µg/kg), inhalation (24 µg/kg), and oral routes (6 mg per kg) to Sprague-Dawley rats weighing between 175 and 250 g, respectively. They noted that while doses in the microgram range were useful for monitoring the urinary and faecal excretion of HEX, much higher doses (about 6 mg/kg in 0.5 ml of corn oil, and with a 4-fold increase in radiocarbon activity) were necessary to obtain levels in the principal organs that could be measured with any precision. Indeed, the doses administered orally were some 250 and 600 times the inhaled and intravenous doses, respectively. In agreement with other researchers, these authors attributed the lack of measurable levels in the organs, following the administration of low doses, to the poor bioavailability of HEX when given by the oral route. The total radiolabel recovery immediately after the administration of the dose was 98.0 ± 5.3% (mean ± S.D.). Rats dosed orally eliminated 2-3 times more of the dose in the faeces than those dosed by the intravenous or inhalation route. A maximum blood level was reached at approximately 2 h after dosing. The peak was broad with similar blood concentrations between 2 and 5 h, perhaps indicating that absorption occurred along the gastrointestinal tract over this period in a quasi-steady state with elimination. Biliary excretion was again confirmed as being greater after oral dosing than after intravenous or inhalation dosing, but it still only accounted for 18% of the administered dose. This observation agreed with previous studies and, more importantly, with the report of Yu & Atallah (1981), who administered comparable dose levels by the oral route. Lawrence & Dorough (1982) also reported that the faecal material contained predominantly polar or unextractable material, as did the bile. These authors considered that this was a clear indication that ^{14}C-HEX was extensively metabolized to polar products by the gut contents, since only approximately 50% of ^{14}C-HEX was recovered when it was added to rat stomach contents that were then immediately extracted with hexane.

A more recent comparative study (El Dareer et al., 1983) essentially confirmed the findings of Yu & Atallah

Kinetics and Metabolism

(1981) and Lawrence & Dorough (1982). Male Fischer-344 rats with an average body weight of 169 g were dosed at a level of 4.1 and 61 mg/kg with approximately 1 ml of a solution of ^{14}C-HEX dissolved in a 1:1:4 mixture of Emulphor EL620, ethanol, and water. Little radioactivity appeared as exhaled ^{14}CO$_2$.

6.1.2 Inhalation

In studies by Dorough (1980) and Lawrence & Dorough (1981, 1982), rats were exposed to ^{14}C-HEX vapour in a specially designed, single animal inhalation exposure system. Each animal was exposed to the vapours in a rodent respirator, with the exhaust vapours from the system passing through a filter pad made from expanded polyurethane foam. The flow rate and concentration of HEX was measured prior to and after passing through the respirator containing the exposed animal. The difference between the amounts of HEX in the input and output was assumed to be equivalent to the retained dose. Rats were exposed for a period of 1 h and received doses in air which ranged from 1.4 to 37.4 mg/kg body weight (Lawrence & Dorough, 1981). Immediately after the 1-h exposure, the recovery of the dose retained by the animal was 91.8 ± 8.5% (mean ± S.D.). Exposed animals were immediately placed in metabolism cages for 72 h, during which time faeces, urine, and expired air were collected. The animals were then killed and certain of their tissues analysed for ^{14}C activity. Less than 1% of the retained radiocarbon was expired during the 24-h period immediately following exposure, and no radiocarbon was detected as ^{14}CO$_2$. Only about 69% of the inhaled dose was recovered, which was much lower than that recovered after intravenous (85%) or oral dosing (82%). Since recovery of the dose immediately after the administration of the inhalation dose was approximately 92%, the reduced recovery during the 72-h post-dosing period led to the speculation that a volatile metabolite was formed during this period, but attempts to collect and identify this metabolite were not successful.

No kinetic parameters were reported in either of the publications by Lawrence & Dorough (1981, 1982), although blood concentration-time data during the 1-h exposure and the following 6 h were presented. Elimination during the subsequent 6 h appeared to relate to a complex pharmacokinetic model with a terminal rate comparable to that reported for the intravenous route, the half-life being approximately 30 h.

The elimination via the bile was relatively low (8%) after inhalation exposure, compared with 13 and 18% after intravenous or oral administration of the same dose (5 µg/kg) (Lawrence & Dorough, 1982). The fraction of the dose recovered in the faeces and urine (23 and 33%, respectively) was about the same as that recovered after the intravenous dose, except that more was recovered in the urine than in the faeces after the inhalation exposure, while the reverse was observed after the intravenous dose.

A comparative study of the uptake, distribution, and elimination of ^{14}C-HEX (El Dareer et al., 1983) confirmed and extended the conclusions reached by Lawrence & Dorough (1981, 1982) concerning pulmonary exposure. Individual Fischer-344 rats weighing between 125 and 190 g (with an average weight of 169 g) were placed in metabolism cages and exposed by inhalation. The dose received by each rat over a 2-h exposure period was calculated from the total amount of radioactivity recovered from the tissues, faeces, urine, and exhaled air. The animal fur was not included. The dose received by the exposed animals was between 1.3 and 1.8 mg/kg body weight. The animals were killed at either 6 or 24 h after they were removed from the inhalation exposure. Whole blood, plasma, liver, kidneys, voluntary muscle (gastrocnemius), subcutaneous fat, brain, skin (ears), and the residual carcass (except for the skin and fur which were discarded) were analysed for ^{14}C activity, as were the urine, faeces, and exhaled air. The principal sites of deposition were the lungs, kidneys, and liver. Only approximately 1% of the radiolabel was identified as ^{14}CO$_2$. No intact HEX was found in any of the tissues; the majority of the radiolabel extracted was polar (water soluble). These findings were similar to those of Lawrence & Dorough (1981, 1982).

6.1.3 Dermal

No studies on the pharmacokinetics or distribution of dermally applied HEX were found in a survey of the pub-

Kinetics and Metabolism

lished literature. Although no qualitative studies or estimates of the uptake of HEX through skin were found, studies have been reported in which discoloration of the skin was observed after the dermal application of HEX (Treon at al., 1955; IRDC, 1972). In these reports, toxic response, leading to death, was observed in several instances, which would suggest that HEX was absorbed transdermally into the systemic circulation.

6.1.4 Comparative studies

Each of the four major studies (Yu & Atallah, 1981; Lawrence & Dorough, 1981, 1982; El Dareer et al., 1983) of the uptake and distribution of HEX involved more than one route of uptake. One objective of each of these studies was to compare the exposure routes. The observations made were as follows:

- The principal routes of excretion were via the urine and faeces. Considerably more of the administered dose was excreted in the faeces after oral administration than after dosing by the intravenous or inhalation route, probably as a consequence of the increased biliary excretion after oral dosing and the interaction or metabolism of the dose by gut and faecal contents. More of the administered dose was excreted in the urine than in the faeces after inhalation exposure, while the reverse was the case after intravenous administration.

- Biliary excretion occurred after administration by each of the three routes. For similar doses, the fraction of the dose eliminated by this route was in the order oral > intravenous > inhalation.

- Comparative distribution to the major organs and tissues is presented in Tables 8, 9, and 10. The principal organs to which HEX was distributed by the systemic circulation were the kidneys and liver. The lungs and trachea contained the highest concentrations of HEX after inhalation exposure.

- There was a significantly higher retention of ^{14}C in the carcass, at 72 h post-dosing, after dosing by the inhalation and intravenous routes than after oral dosing (Table 10).

Table 8. Distribution of radioactivity (expressed as percentage of administered dose) from ^{14}C-HEX in rats dosed by various routes[a]

	Oral dose		Intravenous dose[b]	Inhalation dose	
	Low dose[b] (4.1 mg/kg)	High dose[b] (61 mg/kg)	0.59 mg/kg	Group A[c] (1.0 mg/kg)	Group B[b] (1.4 mg/kg)
Faeces	74.5 ± 2.8	65.3 ± 6.9	34.0 ± 1.0[d]	28.7 ± 4.3	47.5 ± 6.4
Urine	35.5 ± 2.5	28.7 ± 4.2	15.8 ± 1.4	41.0 ± 4.8	40.0 ± 6.6
Tissues	2.4 ± 0.6	2.4 ± 0.1	39.0 ± 1.0	28.9 ± 1.6	11.5 ± 0.8
CO_2	0.8 ± 0.0	0.6 ± 0.0	0.1 ± 0.0	1.4 ± 0.3	1.0 ± 0.5
Other volatile compounds	0.2 ± 0.0	0.3 ± 0.0	0.1 ± 0.0		
Total recovery	118 ± 3.0[e]	97 ± 7.0	89 ± 2.0	100	100

[a] Adapted from: El Dareer et al. (1983). Values represent the mean percentage of dose ± S.D. for three rats.
[b] At 72 h after dosing or exposure.
[c] At 6 h after exposure.
[d] Plus intestinal contents.
[e] For an unexplained reason, the total recovery for this dose was higher than theoretical. If the percent recoveries for this dose are "normalized" to 100%, differences in distribution for the two doses are minimal, indicating that no saturable process is operative in this dose range.

Table 9. Fate of radiocarbon (expressed as percentage of administered dose) after oral, inhalation, and intravenous exposure of rats to ^{14}C-HEX[a]

	Cumulative percent of dose		
	Oral[b]	Intravenous[c]	Inhalation[d]
24-h			
Urine	22.2 ± 1.8	18.3 ± 5.2	29.7 ± 4.5
Faeces	62.2 ± 8.0	21.1 ± 7.1	17.0 ± 7.5
48-h			
Urine	24.0 ± 1.9	20.7 ± 5.6	32.5 ± 5.1
Faeces	67.7 ± 5.1	30.4 ± 1.7	21.0 ± 7.5
72-h			
Urine	24.4 ± 1.9	22.1 ± 5.7	33.1 ± 4.5
Faeces	68.2 ± 5.1	47.4 ± 1.9	23.1 ± 5.7
Body	0.2 ± 0.2	15.7 ± 7.8	12.9 ± 4.7
Total Recovery	92.8 ± 4.7	85.2 ± 4.8	69.1 ± 9.6

[a] Adapted from: Dorough (1980) and Lawrence & Dorough (1982).
[b] Dose (7 µg/kg body weight) administered in 0.5 ml corn oil.
[c] Dose (5 µg/kg body weight) administered in 0.2 ml saline:propylene glycol:ethanol (10:4:1) by injection into the femoral vein.
[d] Doses administered as vapours over a 1-h exposure period to achieve doses of about 24 µg/kg body weight.

6.1.5 In vitro studies

Yu & Atallah (1981) examined the ability of liver, faecal, and gut homogenates to metabolize HEX *in vitro*. In an apparent first-order kinetic process, HEX was metabolized by gut content, faecal, and liver homogenates with half-lives of 10.6, 1.6, and 14.2 h, respectively. When mercuric chloride ($HgCl_2$) was added to the gut and faecal homogenates as a bacteriocide, the half-lives were increased to 17.2 and 6.2 h, respectively, indicating that the gut and faecal flora contributed significantly to the metabolism of HEX. Denaturation of the liver homogenate had virtually no effect on the *in vitro* metabolic rate indicating, perhaps, that there was only limited involvement of liver microsomes or other enzyme-dependent process.

El Dareer et al. (1983) incubated ^{14}C-HEX with homogenates of liver, faeces, and intestinal (large and small)

Table 10. Distribution of HEX equivalents[a] in tissues and excreta of rats 72 h after oral, inhalation, and intravenous exposure to ^{14}C-HEX[b,c]

Sample	Oral dose (6 mg/kg)[d]	Inhaled dose (24 µg/kg)	Intravenous dose (10 µg/kg)
ng/g of tissue			
Trachea	292 ± 170	107.0 ± 65.0	3.3 ± 1.7
Lungs	420 ± 250	71.5 ± 55.2	14.9 ± 1.1
Liver	539 ± 72	3.6 ± 1.9	9.6 ± 1.1
Kidneys	3272 ± 84	29.5 ± 20.2	22.3 ± 0.6
Fat	311 ± 12	2.8 ± 0.4	2.3 ± 0.2
Remaining carcass	63 ± 40	1.3 ± 0.6	0.5 ± 0.1
percentage of dose			
Whole body	2.8 ± 1.1	12.9 ± 4.7	31.0 ± 7.8
Urine	15.3 ± 3.3	33.1 ± 4.5	22.1 ± 5.7
Faeces	63.6 ± 8.5	23.1 ± 5.7	31.4 ± 1.9
Total recovery	81.7 ± 6.7	69.1 ± 9.6	84.6 ± 4.6

[a] One HEX equivalent is defined as the amount of radiolabel equivalent to 1 ng of HEX, based on the specific activity of the dosing solution.
[b] Adapted from: Dorough (1980) and Lawrence & Dorough (1982).
[c] All values are the mean ± S.D. of three replicates.
[d] It should be noted that the oral dose was 250 and 600 times that of the inhaled and intravenous doses, respectively. This was necessary because residues were not detected in individual tissues of animals treated orally at doses of 5-25 µg/kg.

contents, as well as with whole blood and plasma. Samples were taken at 0, 5, and 60 min. The results, presented in Table 11, clearly demonstrated the chemical reactivity of HEX and its ability to bind components of biological material.

6.2 Metabolic transformation

No primary metabolites or conjugates of HEX have been identified. The data available on the pharmacokinetics of HEX after dosing by the oral, inhalation, and dermal routes are presented in sections 6.1.1, 6.1.2, and 6.1.3. In studies by Dorough (1980) and Lawrence & Dorough (1982), the principal routes of excretion were shown to be via the urine and faeces. No unchanged HEX was found in either, indicating that HEX was involved in extensive metabolism.

In studies with rats and mice fed a diet containing 1, 5, or 25 mg ^{14}C-HEX/kg, 63-79% of the consumed HEX was

Table 11. Extractability of ^{14}C-HEX and radioactivity derived from saline and various biological preparations[a]

Preparation	Time (min)	First Extraction Organic[b]	First Extraction Aqueous	Second Extraction Organic	Second Extraction Aqueous	Pellet
Saline	0	99.6 (92.4)	0.4			
	5	99.1 (92.8)	0.9			
	60	98.8 (94.6)	1.2			
Liver	0	55.0 (74.4)	8.0	24.5	1.0	11.6
	5	42.8 (49.7)	15.2	15.0	4.7	22.2
	60	11.1	18.8	5.9	2.4	51.8
Plasma	0	22.2 (61.7)	7.2	50.2	0.8	19.6
	5	19.7 (66.3)	25.0	33.6	2.0	19.6
	60	1.4	43.4	21.	3.9	30.2
Whole blood	0	16.2 (60.4)	3.8	27.9	1.2	50.8
	5	2.8	21.6	13.4	1.6	60.6
	60	0.6	27.4	12.0	1.4	58.6
Faeces	0	90.0 (93.7)	0.6	8.0	0.2	1.2
	5	83.4 (87.8)	0.8	9.0	0.6	6.2
	60	40.5 (61.0)	2.8	31.3	3.0	22.4
Intestinal contents	0	93.7 (94.7)	0.6	4.6	0.2	1.0
	5	82.8 (89.5)	1.6	8.6	1.0	5.9
	60	66.3 (87.0)	4.6	15.4	2.4	11.3

[a] From: El Dareer et al. (1983). Values represent the percentage of the total radioactivity in the respective fraction.
[b] Values in parentheses represent the percentage of the radioactivity in the fraction as HEX.

recovered in the urine and faeces (Dorough, 1979; Dorough & Ranieri, 1984). The extraction characteristics of the radiocarbon compounds in the excreta showed that they were primarily polar metabolites, some of which were transformed to organic-soluble compounds after acid-catalysed hydrolysis.

In a comparative study of the pharmacokinetics of HEX after intravenous or oral dosing at 8.5-25.6 mg/kg (Yu & Atallah, 1981), urinary and faecal metabolites were again characterized as polar because of their poor solubility in organic solvents. No unchanged HEX was found. Only 11% of the ^{14}C content of the excreta was soluble in organic solvents, and a further 32% of the extract was converted to organic-soluble compounds after acid-catalysed hydrolysis. This indicated, perhaps, that metabolite ester conjugates had been formed.

Yu & Atallah (1981) also performed *in vitro* metabolic studies in which they incubated HEX with liver, faecal, and gut-content homogenates (see section 6.1.5).

After Lawrence & Dorough (1982) had dosed rats by the oral, inhalation, and intravenous routes with ^{14}C-labelled HEX at 6 mg/kg, 24 µg/kg and 10 µg/kg, respectively, they found that the faecal and bile contents contained mostly polar metabolites. These authors suggested that HEX was rapidly metabolized to polar products, since only about 50% of the HEX was recovered when it was added to rat gut contents and immediately extracted with n-hexane. In addition, the authors noted that approximately 15.8 ± 4% of the radiolabel that appeared in the faeces within 24 h after dosing was volatile, indicating that a catabolite was probably produced.

El Dareer et al. (1983) dosed rats by the inhalation route so that individual animals received between 1.3 and 1.8 mg/kg body weight over a 2-h exposure period. They were killed 6 or 24 h after removal from exposure. No intact HEX was found in any of the tissues, and the majority of the extractable material was polar (water soluble), in accordance with the findings of Lawrence & Dorough (1981, 1982). As a part of this same study, El Dareer et al. (1983) incubated ^{14}C-HEX with homogenates of liver, faeces, and intestinal (large and small) contents, as well as with whole blood and plasma. These *in vitro* studies

Kinetics and Metabolism

were designed to assess the reactivity and binding characteristics of HEX. The results, presented in Table 8, clearly show chemical lability of HEX and its ability to bind the components of biological material (see section 6.1.2).

Despite these efforts to characterize HEX metabolism, no metabolites were identified. This observation suggests that an attempt to rectify this deficiency would be a high priority.

6.3 Reaction with body components

The toxic mechanisms of hexachlorocyclopentadiene are not well understood. HEX has been shown to react with olefins and other organic molecules such as aromatic compounds. Using the available data, especially those from studies comparing the various routes of exposure, a very general and hypothetical rationale can be developed to suggest possible reactions with body tissue.

The reactivity of HEX shows a high potential for transformation and reaction with other chemicals. Absorption from the gastrointestinal contents is relatively inefficient, probably due to the interaction of HEX with the gastrointestinal contents and metabolism by intestinal flora. The fact that HEX did not appear to be interactive with the gastrointestinal epithelia in the kinetic studies discussed in this chapter was probably due to its dilution in the carrier vehicle, as well as its interaction with, and metabolism by, the gut contents. However, in short-term repeated oral dosing studies (SRI, 1981a,b), at doses of 19 mg/kg or more, inflammation and hyperplasia was noted in the forestomach (see Table 16). In addition, the interaction of HEX after dermal contact was marked by a distinct discoloration of the skin. This suggests a "site of uptake" interaction, probably similar to that observed in the lungs after pulmonary uptake.

During inhalation and the passage of HEX through the lung tissue to reach the systemic circulation, metabolism to water-soluble compounds probably occurs and HEX is eliminated through the kidneys. However, an intravenous dose may be bound unchanged to blood components (e.g., haemoglobin) and remain attached until reaching the liver.

The relatively slow elimination of the radiolabel from the systemic circulation after intravenous dosing with ^{14}C-HEX (approximate terminal half-life of 30 h) suggests a bioaccumulation potential, at least for some of the metabolites, since little HEX appears to remain in the tissues.

Rand et al. (1982b) showed that the cellular level in lung tissue underwent significant changes after HEX inhalation. HEX vapour, administered by the inhalation route, in addition to binding to epithelial lung tissue, was found to bind to the extracellular lining in the lung. Binding to bronchiolar Clara cells, which contribute important materials to the extracellular lining of the peripheral airways, was observed after inhalation exposure in rats and monkeys (Rand et al., 1982a). HEX was also found, in *in vitro* studies, to bind to the components of whole blood, plasma, liver, and faecal homogenates and to gastrointestinal contents (El Dareer et al., 1983). Thus, irrespective of the route of administration, the principal sites of toxic action seem to be the lungs, liver, and kidneys. This observation is supported by the results from the toxicity testing reported in chapter 8.

7. EFFECTS ON ORGANISMS IN THE ENVIRONMENT

7.1 Microorganisms

The effects of HEX on microorganisms have been studied in aqueous and soil systems. Many of the aqueous concentrations used in these experiments exceeded the upper limit of aqueous solubility (0.8-2.1 mg/litre). These concentrations were usually obtained by using an organic solvent vehicle to disperse the chemical in aqueous media. The environmental significance of the results should be interpreted with this aspect in mind.

Cole (1953) inoculated 10 strains of common human and animal pathogens into growth media that contained various concentrations of HEX. The inhibiting concentration, or lowest concentration in which no growth was observed after 96 h of contact, ranged from 1-10 mg HEX/litre. The Addition of 5 or 10 mg HEX/litre to sewage effluent inoculated with *Salmonella typhosa* was found to be more effective than similar concentrations of chlorine in reducing counts of total bacteria, coliforms, and *S. typhosa* (Cole, 1954). Yowell (1951) also reported, in a patent application, that HEX has antibacterial properties; standard phenol coefficients for *Ebertnella typhi (Salmonella typhi)* and *Staphylococcus aureus* were 25 and 33, at 21 and 23 mg HEX/litre, respectively. These findings indicate that concentrations of HEX at or slightly above its aqueous solubility limit are toxic to several types of pathogens.

In contrast, tests with other microorganisms have shown some ability to withstand HEX exposure. Twenty-three strains of organisms (type unspecified), when added to aqueous media containing HEX at 1000 mg/litre, were able to metabolize the compound to a varying degree. Analysis of the medium after 14 days indicated a HEX removal of 2-76%, depending on the organism used (Thuma et al., 1978).

Rieck (1977a) found no effects on natural populations of bacteria, actinomycetes, or fungi after a 24-day incubation of a sandy loam soil treated with 1 or 10 mg HEX/kg dry weight. It was concluded that no significant detrimental effects on microbial populations would result from contamination of soils with these levels of HEX.

The effects of HEX on three ecologically important microbial processes have been reported (Butz & Atallah, 1980). Results on cellulose degradation by the fungus *Trichoderma longibrachiatum* indicated that a suspension of HEX inhibited cellulose degradation at a concentration of 1 mg/litre or more in a liquid medium. The calculated 7-day EC_{50} was 1.1 mg/litre. Extrapolations for 1- and 3-day EC_{50} values were both reported to be 0.2 mg/litre. The decrease in toxicity over the 7-day period was attributed to adaptation by *T. longibrachiatum*.

HEX inhibited anaerobic sulfate reduction by the bacterium *Desulfovibrio desulfuricans* when HEX was present in suspension in a liquid medium. After a 3-h contact period, growth inhibition was observed at HEX concentrations of 10-100 mg/litre, and there was no growth at 500 or 1000 mg/litre. Similarly, growth inhibition was observed at 1 and 10 mg/litre after a 24-h contact period, and there was no growth at 50-1000 mg/litre. HEX was considered to be slightly toxic to *D. desulfuricans* (Butz & Atallah, 1980).

The third part of the study by these investigators (Butz & Atallah, 1980) focused on the effects of HEX on urea ammonification by a mixed microbial culture in moist soil. The results indicated that HEX concentrations of 1-100 mg/kg (dry weight) were not toxic to soil organisms responsible for urea ammonification. The EC_{50} increased from 104 mg/kg at day 1 to 1374 mg/kg at day 14. The authors suggested that the low toxicity and its decrease over time in this experiment may have been due to adsorption of the toxicant onto soil particles, as well as to potential adaptation by the organism. Adsorption onto soil particles may also account for the lack of toxicity in the study of Rieck (1977a).

Walsh (1981) reported unpublished data on the effects of HEX on four species of marine algae, obtained according to the method described by Walsh & Alexander (1980). The 7-day EC_{50} was calculated as the concentration that caused a 50% decrease in growth compared with the control, as estimated by absorbance at 525 nm. The 7-day EC_{50} values reported indicated a wide range of susceptibility among the species tested. *Isochrysis galbana* and *Skeletonema costatum* were the most susceptible species, the average 7-day EC_{50} values being about 3.5 and 6.6 µg per litre, respectively. The average value for *Porphyridium cruentum* was 30 µg/litre, while that for *Dunaliella tertiolecta* was 100 µg/litre. Other tests with *S. costatum* indicated that the direct algicidal effect of HEX was less pronounced than its effect on growth. After 48 h of exposure to HEX at 25 µg/litre, mortality, as indicated by staining and cell enumeration, was only 4% (Walsh, 1983).

7.2 Aquatic organisms

7.2.1 Freshwater aquatic life

Several studies are available on the effects resulting from exposure of freshwater aquatic life to various concentrations of HEX.

Results from acute toxicity tests with HEX have been reported for a number of freshwater fish species (Table 12). The 96-h LC_{50} value for fathead minnow larvae in a flow-through test with measured toxicant concentration was 7 µg/litre (Spehar et al., 1977, 1979). Values obtained for adult fathead minnows in static tests with unmeasured toxicant concentrations ranged from 59 to 180 µg/litre (Henderson, 1956; Buccafusco & LeBlanc, 1977). Reported 96-h values for goldfish, channel catfish, and bluegills were also within this range (Buccafusco & LeBlanc, 1977; Podowski & Khan, 1979; Khan et al., 1981).

Sinhaseni et al. (1982) reported the biological effects of HEX on rainbow trout *(Salmo gairdneri)* exposed to 130 µg HEX/litre in a non-recirculating flow-through chamber. Oxygen consumption, measured polarographically, increased by 193% within 80 min and then gradually decreased until the fish died (after approximately 5 h). Vehicle controls showed no effects after 76 h of exposure. When added to normal trout mitochondria, HEX increased basal oxygen consumption. The authors concluded that HEX uncoupled oxidative phosphorylation.

Sinhaseni et al. (1983) continued their research on the respiratory effects of HEX on intact rainbow trout.

Table 12. Acute toxicity data for freshwater species exposed to HEX

Species	Method[a]	LC$_{50}$ (μg/litre)[b]			Acute no-effect concentration (μg/litre)	Comments	Reference
		24-h	48-h	96-h			
Cladoceran *Daphnia magna*	S,U	93.0 (78.9-109.6)	52.2 (44.8-60.9)	ND	32	17 °C, soft water	Vilkas (1977)
Cladoceran *Daphnia magna*	S,U	130 (68-260)	39 (30-52)	ND	18	22 °C, soft water	Buccafusco & Leblanc (1977)
Fathead minnow (larvae, < 0.1 g) *Pimephales promelas*	FT,M	NR	NR	7.0	3.7	25 °C, soft water	Spehar et al. (1977, 1979)
Fathead minnow (1-1.5 g) *Pimephales promelas*	S,U	115 93 75	110 78 59	104 78 59	NR NR NR	Hard water, acetone soln. Soft water, acetone soln. Hard water, emulsion (no acetone)	Henderson (1956)
Fathead minnow (0.72 g) *Pimephales promelas*	S,U	240 (170-320)	210 (180-250)	180 (160-220)	87	22 °C, soft water	Buccafusco & Leblanc (1977)
Goldfish *Carassius auratus*	NR	NR	NR	78	NR	No details given	Podowski & Khan (1979)
Channel catfish (2.1 g) *Ictalurus punctatus*	S,U	190 (140-250)	150 (130-180)	97 (81-120)	56	22 °C, soft water	Buccafusco & Leblanc (1977)
Bluegill (0.45 g) *Lepomis macrochirus*	S,U	170 (140-210)	150 (120-180)	130 (110-170)	65	22 °C, soft water	Buccafusco & Leblanc (1977)

[a] S = static, FT = flow-through, U = unmeasured concentrations, M = measured concentrations.
[b] Numbers in parentheses show 95% confidence interval. ND = Not determined. NR = Not reported.

Acclimated rainbow trout were exposed to 130 µg HEX/litre in a flow-through well-water circuit, which was designed to allow measurements of oxygen consumption in fish. Again, HEX increased oxygen consumption rates (186 ± 24%), the maximum rates being nearly the same as in the previous experiment (approximately 84 min). The oxygen consumption decreased until death (after approximately 6.5 h). Control trout, exposed to the same concentration of the vehicle (acetone) used to disperse HEX, showed no changes. The authors reported profound respiratory stimulation, and HEX appeared to uncouple oxidative phosphorylation. Sinhaseni et al. (1983) postulated that HEX intoxication in the intact animal may be due to increased oxygen consumption and impaired oxidative ATP synthesis resulting from the mitochondrial uncoupling action of HEX.

Spehar et al. (1977, 1979) conducted 30-day early-life stage flow-through toxicity tests with fathead minnows (*Pimephales promelas*) using measured concentrations and 1-day-old larvae. The 96-h LC_{50} value was 7 µg/litre. The 96-h mortality data indicated a sharp toxicity threshold, such that 94% survival was observed at 3.7 µg per litre, 70% at 7.3 µg/litre, and 2% at 9.1 µg/litre. At the end of the 30-day exposure period, mortality was only slightly higher, with 90% survival at 3.7 µg/litre, 66% at 7.3 µg/litre, and 0% at 9.1 µg/litre. These results indicated that the median lethal threshold, the lowest concentration causing 50% mortality, was reached within 4 days. In addition, the HEX residues found in fathead minnows at the end of the 30-day tests were low (< 0.1 µg/g), and a BCF value of < 11 was reported (Spehar et al., 1979). The authors concluded that the toxicity data and the BCF values indicated that HEX was non-cumulative in fish, i.e. it did not bioconcentrate in fish as a result of continuous low-level exposure to HEX. The growth rate of surviving larvae, measured in terms of both body length and weight, did not decrease significantly at any of the concentrations tested, compared with the controls. This was true even at 7.3 µg/litre, a level greater than the calculated LC_{50} value. Based on these toxicity and growth data, Spehar et al. (1977, 1979) concluded that 3.7 µg/litre is the highest concentration of HEX that produces no adverse effects on fathead minnow larvae. No other chronic toxicity data for any freshwater species are available.

7.2.2 Marine and estuarine aquatic life

Among marine invertebrates, the 96-h LC_{50} values for HEX range from 7 to 371 µg/litre (Table 13) (US EPA, 1980a). Except where indicated, these results were obtained from static tests with nominal concentrations of HEX. The highest LC_{50} by far was for the polychaete *Neanthes arenaceodentata*, which is an infaunal organism living in the sediment. The two shrimp species tested were more sensitive to HEX by a factor of 10 or more.

Table 13. Acute toxicity data on estuarine marine organisms exposed to HEX[a]

Species	Method[b]	Salinity (°/∞)	96-h LC_{50}[c] (µg/litre)
Polychaete *Neanthes arenaceodentata*	S,U	28	371 (297-484)
Grass shrimp *Palaemonetes pugio*	S,U	22	42 (36-50)
Mysid shrimp *Mysidopis bahia*	S,U	24	32 (27-37)
Mysid shrimp *Mysidopsis bahia*	FT,U	24	12 (10-13)
Mysid shrimp *Mysidopsis bahia*	FT,M	24	7 (6-8)
Pinfish *Lagodon rhomboides*	S,U	22	48 (41-58)
Spot *Leiostomus xanthurus*	S,U	22	37 (30-42)
Sheepshead minnow *Cyprinodon variegatus*	S,U	24	45 (34-61)

[a] Adapted from: US EPA (1980a) and Mayer (1987).
[b] S = static; FT = flow-through; U = unmeasured concentrations; M = measured concentrations.
[c] Numbers in parentheses show 95% confidence interval.

The static LC_{50} value reported by US EPA (1980a) for the grass shrimp, *Palaemonetes pugio*, was slightly higher than that for the mysid shrimp, *Mysidopsis bahia* (Table

Effects on Organisms in the Environment

13). However, the LC_{50} for the mysid shrimp was considerably lower in a flow-through test than in the static test.

Similarly, the LC_{50} value was lower when calculated from actual measurements of HEX concentrations in the test solutions (measured concentration) than when calculated according to the concentrations based on amounts originally added to test solutions (nominal concentrations).

The acute toxicity values for HEX were similar for each of three estuarine and marine fish species tested (US EPA, 1980a). The static 96-h LC_{50} values based on unmeasured concentrations for spot, sheepshead minnow, and pinfish varied only between 37 and 48 µg/litre (Table 13).

7.3 Terrestrial organisms and wildlife

In a USA patent application, HEX was reported to be nontoxic to plants in concentrations at which it was an effective fungicide (Yowell, 1951). Test solutions were prepared by adding HEX at various proportions to attaclay and a wetting agent, and they were then mixed with water. The concentrations of HEX applied to plants as an aqueous spray were 0.1, 0.2, 0.5, and 1.0%. Slight injury (unspecified) to *Coleus blumei* was reported at 1.0% HEX, but lower concentrations were not harmful. Similarly, HEX was added to horticultural spray oil and an emulsifier at various proportions and then mixed with water. The concentations of HEX in the prepared spray were 0.25 and 0.5%. No injury to *C. blumei* was observed at these concentrations. No data are available concerning the effects of HEX on amphibians, reptiles, birds, or mammals other than those routinely used in laboratory testing.

7.4 Population and ecosystem effects

The ecological effects of HEX have not been studied at the ecosystem, population, or community levels.

8. EFFECTS ON EXPERIMENTAL ANIMALS AND *IN VITRO* TEST SYSTEMS

8.1 Acute toxicity studies

8.1.1 Acute oral, inhalation, and dermal toxicity

The data from acute toxicity studies using HEX are summarized in Table 14. Caution should be exercised in comparing the various studies. The acute toxicity (LD_{50} and LC_{50}) may be affected not only by the species and age of the animals used in the experimental tests, but also by the strain. In addition, the purity of the compound and the nature of the contaminants may affect the toxicity, as can the experimental method and the vehicle used. These details (when specified by the researchers) have been summarized in the table.

For the rat, oral LD_{50} values ranged from 425 to 926 mg/kg for males, and from 315 to 926 mg/kg for females. Values for mice and rabbits were within the same range.

Acute inhalation experiments involved exposure durations from 3.5 to 4 h, and LC_{50} values for male rats ranged from 18.1 to 35.0 mg/m^3 (1.6 to 3.1 ppm) and for female rats from 35.0 to 40.0 mg/m^3 (3.1 to 3.5 ppm). The mouse, rabbit, and guinea-pig values ranged from 23.7 to 80.2 mg/m^3 (2.1 to 7.1 ppm).

There are few data available on dermal toxicity. LD_{50} values of < 200 mg/kg in male rabbits and 340-780 mg/kg in females have been reported.

In spite of variations in LD_{50} values in the different studies, these data suggest that HEX is moderately toxic when administered orally. The acute toxicity of HEX by the dermal route is quite similar to its acute oral toxicity. HEX is much more toxic by the inhalation route of exposure than by the dermal or oral routes.

8.1.2 Eye and skin irritation

IRDC (1972) tested HEX for eye irritation by instilling 0.1 ml HEX into the eyes of New Zealand white rabbits

Table 14. Acute toxicity studies of HEX

Species (strain) age	Route (vehicle)	Results[a]	Reference
Oral LD_{50}			
Rat (unspecified) young adult	oral gavage (5% solution of peanut oil)	M: 510 mg/kg F: 690 mg/kg	Treon et al. (1955)
Rat (Charles River CD) young adult	oral gavage (corn oil)	M + F: 926 mg/kg	IDRC (1968)
Rat (Sprague-Dawley) young adult		M + F: 651 mg/kg	Dorough (1979)
Rat (Fischer-344) weanling	oral gavage (corn oil)	M: 425 mg/kg F: 315 mg/kg	SRI (1980a)
Mouse (unspecified)		M + F: 600 mg/kg	Dorough (1979)
Mouse ($B6C3F_1$) weanling	oral gavage (corn oil)	M + F: 680 mg/kg	SRI (1980a)
Rabbit (Albino, strain unspecified) adult	oral gavage (5% peanut oil)	F: 640 mg/kg	Treon et al. (1955)
Dermal LD_{50}			
Rabbit (unspecified) adult	skin painted	F: 780 mg/kg	Treon et al. (1955)
Rabbit (unspecified) adult	skin painted	M: < 200 mg/kg F: 340 mg/kg	IDRC (1972)
Inhalation LC_{50}			
Rat (Carworth) young adult	inhalation	3.5-h LC_{50} M + F: 35.0 mg/m^3 (3.1 ppm)	Treon et al. (1955)
Rat (Sprague-Dawley) young adult	inhalation	4.0-h LC_{50} M: 18.1 mg/m^3 (1.6 ppm) F: 39.6 mg/m^3 (3.5 ppm)	Rand et al. (1982a)
Mouse (unspecified) young adult	inhalation	3.5-h LC_{50} M + F: 23.7 mg/m^3 (2.1 ppm)	Treon et al. (1955)
Rabbit (unspecified) adult	inhalation	3.5-h LC_{50} F: 58.8 mg/m^3 (5.2 ppm)	Treon et al. (1955)
Guinea-pig (unspecified) adult	inhalation	3.5-h LC_{50} M + F: 80.2 mg/m^3 (7.1 ppm)	Treon et al. (1955)

[a] M = male; F = female.

for 5 min or 24 h before washing. All the rabbits died on or before the ninth day of the observation period. Treon et al. (1955) reported HEX to be a primary skin irritant in rabbits (strain unspecified) at a dose level of 250 mg/kg, and IRDC (1972) reported HEX to be a dermal irritant because of the oedema that appeared after application of 0.5 ml HEX. In this study, intense discoloration of the skin was noted. In the study of Treon et al. (1955), monkeys (strain unspecified) were also tested, and discoloration of the skin was noted even at low doses (0.05 ml of 10% HEX) (Table 15).

Table 15. Primary eye and dermal irritation

Study	Species (strain) age	Results	Reference
Primary eye irritation	Rabbit (New Zealand white) adult	Severe eye irritant (0.1 ml for 5 min or 24 h); all died by day 9 of study	IRDC (1972)
Primary dermal irritation	Rabbit (unspecified) adult	Moderate skin irritant (250 mg/kg); one application	Treon et al. (1955)
Primary dermal irritation	Rabbit (New Zealand white) adult	Severe skin irritant (200 mg/kg); all males died	IRDC (1972)
Primary dermal irritation	Monkey (unspecified) adult	Mild skin discoloration (0.05 ml of 10% HEX solution)	Treon et al. (1955)

Shell Research Limited conducted a study of the skin-sensitizing potential of 98.8% pure HEX (Shell Research Limited, 1982). Guinea-pigs (310-370g) were placed at random into single sex groups of 10 animals and housed in groups of five animals. Range-finding tests were conducted to determine the concentrations of test material to be used for intradermal induction, topical induction, and topical challenge. Two male and two female guinea-pigs were injected intradermally on each side of the midline with 0.1 ml of several dilutions (0.5, 1, 5, and 10 mg HEX per ml HEX corn oil). Filter paper patches with 0.3 ml of a 1% or 2% dilution of test material in corn oil were applied to two other groups. On the basis of the results of the range-finding studies, the following tests and HEX concentrations were selected for use: intradermal induction, 0.5 mg/litre; topical induction, 20.5 mg/litre; and topical challenge, 10 mg/ml (all in corn oil). In the sensitizing test, all four animals given an intradermal injection of 0.5 mg HEX/ml suffered necrosis, while topical applications at 10 or 20.5 mg/litre produced slight redness or no difference from surrounding skin. However, all 20 test animals showed positive responses 24 and 48 h after removal of the challenge patches. The researchers concluded that HEX is a skin sensitizer.

8.2 Short-term exposure

8.2.1 Oral

In a range-finding study using groups of five male and five female Fischer-344 rats, there were no deaths when 12 doses of 25, 50, or 100 mg/kg were given in 16 days (SRI, 1980b). With the same dosing schedule, one out of five males and four out of five females died when the dose was 200 mg/kg, and five out of five males and four out of five females died when the dose was 400 mg/kg. In the same study, $B6C3F_1$ mice died when given doses of 400 or 800 mg/kg, but not when given doses of 50, 100, or 200 mg/kg. Both rats and mice exhibited pathological changes of the stomach wall at all but the lowest dose level.

The short-term toxicity of HEX is summarized in Table 16. These short-term toxicity studies on $B6C3F_1$ mice and Fischer-344 rats were conducted by SRI (1981a,b) under contract with the National Toxicology Program (NTP), and the results were reported by Abdo et al. (1984). In the mouse study (SRI, 1981a), HEX (94.3-97.4% pure) in corn oil was administered by gavage at dose levels of 19, 38, 75, 150, and 300 mg/kg to 10 mice of each sex, 5 days/week for 13 weeks (91 days). At the highest dose level (300 mg/kg), all 10 male mice died by day 8 and three females died by day 14. In female mice, the liver was enlarged. Toxic nephrosis in females at doses of 75 mg/kg or more was characterized by distensions in the proximal convoluted tubules, with basophilia in the inner cortical zone and cytoplasmic vacuolization. However, male mice administered 75 mg/kg or more did not show these effects. Dose

Table 16. Short-term toxicity of HEX

Study	Species	Dose	Results	Effects at LOEL or lowest dose	Reference
90-day feeding study	rat	10, 19, 38, 75, and 150 mg/kg (by gavage)	NOAEL: 10 mg/kg LOEL: 19 mg/kg	lesions of forestomach in female rats at 19 mg/kg	SRI (1981b)
14-week inhalation study	rat	0.11, 0.56, and 0.226 mg/m^3 (5 days/week)	NOEL: 0.226 mg/m^3 LOEL: NE	no statistically significant effects	Rand et al. (1982a)
14-week inhalation study	monkey	0.11, 0.56, and 0.226 mg/m^3 (5 days/week)	NOEL: 0.2 ppm LOEL: NE	no effects noted	Alexander et al. (1980)

NE = not established.
NOAEL = no-observed-adverse-effect level.
NOEL = no-observed-effect level.
LOEL = lowest-observed-effect level.

levels of 38 mg/kg or more caused lesions in the forestomach, including ulceration in both males and females, as well as increased kidney and liver weights. The no-observed-adverse-effect level (NOAEL) in mice was 19 mg/kg and the lowest-observed-adverse-effect level (LOAEL) was 38 mg/kg.

In the rat study (SRI, 1981b), HEX in corn oil was administered by gavage at dose levels of 10, 19, 38, 75, and 150 mg/kg to groups of 10 male and female F-344 rats. At 38 mg/kg or more, mortality and toxic nephrosis were observed in both males and females. The male rats treated with 19 mg/kg showed no significant effects, but female rats had lesions in the forestomach. Similar lesions were observed in males given 38 mg/kg or more. There was a dose-related depression of body weight gain (relative to the controls) and female rats had increased kidney and liver weights. The NOAEL in rats was 10 mg/kg, and the lowest-observed-effect level (LOEL) was 19 mg/kg.

A summary of the results of these two experiments appears in Table 17.

8.2.2 Short-term inhalation toxicity

Rand et al. (1982a) conducted a range-finding study in which groups of 10 male and 10 female Sprague-Dawley rats were exposed to atmospheres of 0.25, 1.24, or 5.65 mg HEX/m^3 (0.022, 0.11, or 0.5 ppm), 6 h/day, 5 days/week for a total of 10 exposures. Nine male rats and one female rat exposed to 5.65 mg/m^3 were moribund after five to seven exposures. These rats had dark red eyes, laboured breathing, and pale extremities. There were no mortalities in the other exposure groups. However, the males in the medium- and high-dose groups lost weight during the study and reduced mean liver weights and pathology were noted. The NOAEL for HEX exposure in this study was 0.25 mg/m^3 and the LOEL was 1.24 mg/m^3.

Fourteen-week inhalation studies have been carried out on rats and monkeys (Alexander et al., 1980; Rand et al., 1982a,b) and the results are summarized in Table 16. Groups of 40 male and 40 female Sprague-Dawley rats weighing 160-224 g and groups of 12 Cynomolgus monkeys weighing 1.5-2.5 kg were exposed to HEX, 6 h/day, 5 days

Table 17. Toxicological parameters for mice and rats administered technical grade HEX in corn oil by gavage for 91 days[a]

Species (strain)	Sex	Dose (mg/kg)	Mortality	Relative weight gain[b]	Forestomach inflammation	Forestomach hyperplasia	Toxic nephrosis
Mice (B6C3F$_1$)	male	0	1/10		0/10	0/10	0/10
		19	0/10	+ 36%	0/10	0/10	0/10
		38	0/10	+ 9%	2/10	2/10	0/10
		75	0/10	- 9%	7/10	8/10	0/10
		150	0/10	- 45%	7/10	9/10	0/10
		300	10/10		7/10	8/10	0/10
Mice (B6C3F$_1$)	female	0	0/10		0/10	0/10	0/10
		19	0/10	+ 13%	0/10	0/10	0/10
		38	0/10	- 13%	2/9	2/9	0/9
		75	0/10	- 13%	6/10	9/10	10/10
		150	0/10	- 25%	10/10	10/10	10/10
		300	3/10	- 38%	7/9	9/9	7/10
Rats (F-344)	male	0	3/10		0/10	0/10	0/10
		10	1/10	- 4%	0/10	0/10	0/10
		19	1/10	- 8%	0/10	0/10	0/10
		38	1/10	- 20%	4/10	5/10	10/10
		75	3/10	- 49%	9/10	9/10	9/10
		150	7/10	- 57%	8/9	8/9	8/10
Rats (F-344)	female	0	1/10		0/10	0/10	0/10
		10	2/10	0%	0/10	0/10	0/10
		19	1/10	+ 4%	2/10	2/10	0/10
		38	1/10	- 5%	2/10	5/10	10/10
		75	3/10	- 30%	9/10	9/10	10/10
		150	5/10	- 33%	9/10	9/10	10/10

[a] From: SRI (1981a,b).
[b] Relative weight gain was calculated as follows:

$$\frac{\text{Dose group value - control group value}}{\text{Control group value}} \times 100$$

per week, for 14 weeks. Levels of exposure were 0, 0.11, 0.56, and 2.26 mg/m^3 (0, 0.01, 0.05, and 0.20 ppm). In monkeys, there were no mortalities, adverse clinical signs, weight gain changes, pulmonary function changes, eye lesions, haematological changes, clinical chemistry abnormalities, or histopathological abnormalities at any dose level tested. Thus, the NOEL for monkeys was at least 2.26 mg/m^3 for this exposure period, but the LOEL was not established. Male rats had a transient appearance of dark-red eyes at 0.56 and 2.26 mg/m^3. At 12 weeks, there were marginal but not statistically significant increases in haemoglobin concentration and erythrocyte count in males exposed to 0.11 mg/m^3, females exposed to 0.56 mg/m^3, and males and females exposed to 2.26 mg/m^3. There were small but not statistically significant changes in mean liver weight of all groups of treated rats and similar changes in the kidneys of all treated males. No treatment-related abnormalities in gross pathology or histopathology were observed. On this basis, the NOEL in rats was 2.26 mg/m^3, but the LOEL was not established.

In a further study by Rand et al. (1982b), no ultrastructural changes were observed in monkeys that could be attributed to the inhalation of HEX vapour. Exposure was identical to that of the previous study (Rand et al., 1982a). There was a statistically significant ($P < 0.01$) increase in the mean number of electronlucent inclusions in the apex and base of the Clara cells in exposed animals, as compared with the controls. According to some researchers (Evans et al., 1978), Clara cells respond to injury by regression to a more primitive cell type. Rand et al. (1982b) noted that some of the ultrastructural changes in the exposed animals resembled those of the Evans study. It is not known what effect these changes might cause. The Clara cell contributes important materials to the extracellular lining of the peripheral airways, and if this effect of HEX vapour causes a change in the content of the contributed material, then the extracellular lining may be altered and breathing may be subsequently impaired (Rand et al., 1982b). This observation of lung effects coincides with those of other researchers (Dorough, 1979, 1980; Lawrence & Dorough, 1981, 1982). Furthermore, in inhalation studies with HEX occasional statistically significant increases in the haemoglobin level and red blood cell counts of rats have been noted, which may be manifestations of the impairment of respiratory functions.

In 1984, the US National Toxicology Program (NTP) completed a short-term, 90-day HEX inhalation study on B6C3F$_1$ mice and F-344 rats (NTP, 1984a,b). In the basic study, ten rats and ten mice of each sex were placed at random into five exposure and control groups. The rats and mice were exposed to nominal concentrations of 0.45, 1.70, 4.52, 11.3, or 22.6 mg/m^3 (0.04, 0.15, 0.4, 1.0, or 2.0 ppm) for 6 h/day, 5 days/week for 13 weeks. In the female mouse study, 6 out of 10 of the control animals died, while none of the animals in the male control population died. The six animal deaths in week 7 were attributed to a defective feeder insert. Mortality in both the rats and mice was high in the two highest-dose groups; all rats and mice in these groups died in the first five weeks of the study. Posterior paresis and listlessness were observed in mice at 4.52 and 11.3 mg/m^3. Compound-related histopathological alterations were observed in the respiratory tracts of male and female mice exposed to 1.7 mg/m^3 or more. These changes included: necrosis, acute and chronic inflammation, hyperplasia or squamous metaplasia of the nasal, laryngeal, tracheal, bronchial, and bronchiolar epithelia of the affected animals. No compound-related effects were observed in mice at the lowest dose, and so this level could be considered the NOEL (NTP, 1984a).

Clinical signs resulting from HEX exposure included posterior paresis in all rats exposed to 1.7 mg/m^3 or more, listlessness in all rats exposed to 4.52 mg/m^3 or more, and eye irritation and respiratory distress in all rats exposed to 11.3 mg/m^3 or more. As in the case of mice, HEX caused significant histological alterations in the respiratory tracts of rats at the two highest doses. Changes of a less-marked degree were observed in the respiratory tracts of rats receiving 4.52 mg/m^3. No compound-related changes were seen in any organ of male and female rats exposed to the lowest dose, and so this level could be considered the NOEL. In addition, compound-related effects of a secondary stress-related nature were seen in a number of other organs of rats of both sexes at

Effects on Experimental Animals and In Vitro Test Systems

the two highest doses. These includes lymphoid depletion of the spleen and thymus, degeneration of the seminiferous tubules and decreased lytoplasmic vacuolization of the adrenal cortex.

Some basic clinical pathology and histopathology examinations were undertaken simultaneously in both studies (NTP, 1984a,b). All effects were similar to those noted in the previous toxicity studies. In the rat study (NTP, 1984b), HEX nephrotoxicity was examined in more depth. HEX was not found to be nephrotoxic at these exposure levels, nor did it appear that it was myelotoxic.

8.2.3 Short-term dermal toxicity

No short-term dermal toxicity studies are available.

8.3 Long-term exposure

8.3.1 Long-term oral toxicity

No long-term oral toxicity studies have been reported.

8.3.2 Long-term inhalation toxicity

In view of the absence of long-term studies on the inhalation of HEX, the following studies were examined. Treon et al. (1955) exposed guinea-pigs, rabbits, rats, and mice to a HEX (89.5% pure) concentration of 3.73 mg/m^3 (0.33 ppm), 7 h/day, 5 days/week, for 25-30 exposure days. The guinea-pigs survived 30 exposures, whereas rats and mice did not survive five exposures, and four out of six rabbits did not survive 25 exposures. Using a lower concentration of 1.70 mg/m^3 (0.15 ppm), guinea-pigs, rabbits, and rats survived 150 7-h exposures over a 7-month period. This level was too high to conduct a long-term study in mice since four out of five animals did not survive. The rats, guinea-pigs, and rabbits tolerated 1.7 mg/m^3 and did not exhibit any treatment-related effects. Thus, the NOEL for rats, guinea-pigs, and rabbits was 1.7 mg/m^3 over the 7-month period. Due to the high mortality, a NOEL for mice could not be established.

A long-term (30 weeks) inhalation study in rats with technical grade HEX (96% pure with hexachlorobuta-1,3-

diene and octachlorocyclopentene as impurities) was conducted by the Shell Toxicology Laboratory (D.G. Clark et al., 1982). Four groups of eight male and eight female Wistar albino rats were exposed to HEX at nominal concentrations of 0, 0.56, 1.13, and 5.65 mg/m^3 (0, 0.05, 0.1, and 0.5 ppm), 6 h/day, 5 days/week, for 30 weeks and were observed for a 14-week recovery period without HEX exposure. At the highest dose level, four males and two females died. In males, there was depressed body weight gain at the highest dose, relative to controls, beginning at 7 weeks of exposure and persisting throughout the remainder of the study. Females in the two highest-dose groups had lower body weights at the end of the recovery period than did the controls. At the highest dose, there were pulmonary degenerative changes, ranging from epithelial hyperplasia and oedema to epithelial ulceration and necrosis, in both sexes, the males being affected more severely. There were also mild degenerative changes in the liver (bile duct hyperplasia and inflammatory cell infiltration) and kidneys (protein casts in tubules and pigmented cortical tubules) in a few rats, and kidney weights were significantly increased in the females at 30 weeks. After 30 weeks of study, no biologically significant toxicity was noted in animals that were exposed to 0.56 or 1.13 mg/m^3. Thus, the NOEL in rats exposed to HEX vapour in this study (6 h/day, 5 days/week, for 30 weeks) was 0.56 mg/m^3, and the LOEL was 1.13 mg/m^3.

A long-term inhalation study by the National Toxicology Program started in January 1986. The animal exposure has been completed and results will be published as soon as the pathology review is completed.

8.3.3 Long-term dermal toxicity

No long-term dermal toxicity studies have been reported.

8.3.4 Principal effects and target organs

Repeated exposure of several animal species to levels of HEX vapour in the range of 1.13 to 2.26 mg/m^3 (0.1-0.2 ppm) has been found to cause pulmonary degenerative changes (Treon et al., 1955; D.G. Clark et al., 1982; Rand et al., 1982a,b). In addition, Treon et al. (1955) reported diffuse degeneration of the brain, heart, and adrenal glands and necrosis of the liver and kidney tubules, together with severe pulmonary hyperaemia and oedema. In many instances, acute bronchitis and interstitial pneumonitis also occurred. Necrosis of the epithelium of the primary, secondary, and tertiary bronchi was observed. At later stages, reacting inflammatory cells migrated into the wall and the mucosa of the bronchi and alveoli. In rabbits, the walls of the alveoli were covered by a hyaline or fibrinoid membrane. Possibly, some of the changes found by Treon et al. (1955) were caused by impurities in the HEX preparation. Acute exposure by the oral and dermal routes also affects the respiratory system (Kommineni, 1978; SRI, 1980a). Death from acute exposure by any tested route seemed to be associated with respiratory failure (Lawrence & Dorough, 1982).

There are insufficient data to identify the site that is the most sensitive to prolonged, repeated exposure to HEX. In comparing routes of administration, researchers found that damage to the lungs occurred regardless of which route was used (Lawrence & Dorough, 1982). When HEX is administered orally to animals, the kidneys may be the most sensitive site, since short-term dosing of rats and mice was found to cause nephrosis, especially in females (SRI, 1981a,b). Although the oral route may not be a significant route of exposure for human beings, the fact that the kidneys are a possible target organ in short-term exposure indicates that low-level, prolonged systemic exposure from any ambient route may affect the kidneys. The liver has also been shown, in several of the laboratory studies, to be affected by HEX.

The available literature does not cite any single mechanism to explain HEX toxicity. HEX vapour irritates the respiratory tract, leading to death by respiratory failure after bronchopneumonia (D.G. Clark et al., 1982). The degenerative changes that have been observed in the liver and kidneys are mild and unlikely to contribute to the chemical's lethality (NAS, 1978; SRI, 1980a,b).

The difficulty in studying HEX because of its high reactivity and volatility has also created problems in identifying its metabolites. Several questions remain as to whether the same metabolites are formed after various routes of exposure and whether it is the administered HEX or its metabolites that cause the lung injuries seen with various dosing regimens. Furthermore, the strong ability of HEX to interact with other compounds, especially organic molecules, can lead to many other effects, such as haemoglobin binding. Little is known about the interactions of HEX with other chemicals in animal or human tissue.

8.4 Developmental and reproductive toxicity

The teratogenic potential of HEX has been evaluated in pregnant Charles River CD-1 rats that were administered HEX (98.25%) in corn oil, by gastric intubation, at dose levels of 3, 10, and 30 mg/kg per day from days 6 to 15 of gestation. A control group received the vehicle (corn oil) at a dose volume of 10 ml/kg per day. All the rats survived, and there was no difference in mean maternal body weight gain between the dosed groups and controls. There were no differences in the mean number of implantations, corpora lutea, live fetuses, mean fetal body weights, or male/female sex ratios among any of the groups, and there were no statistical differences in malformation or developmental variations, compared with the controls, when external, soft tissue, and skeletal examinations were performed (IRDC, 1978).

Murray et al. (1980) evaluated the teratogenic potential of HEX (98%) in CF-1 mice and New Zealand white rabbits. Mice were dosed at 0, 5, 25, or 75 mg HEX/kg per day by gavage during days 6-15 of gestation, while rabbits received the same dose during days 6-18 of gestation. The fertility of the treated mice and rabbits was not significantly different from that of the control groups. In the mice, there was no evidence of maternal toxicity, embryotoxicity, or teratogenic effects. A total of 249-374 fetuses (22-33 litters) was examined in each dose group. In rabbits, maternal toxicity was noted at a dose level of 75 mg/kg (diarrhoea, weight loss, and mortality), but there was no evidence of maternal toxicity at the lower levels. There were no embryotoxic effects at any dose level. Although there was a two-fold increase over controls in the proportion of fetuses with 13 ribs at 75 mg/kg, this was considered to be a minor skeletal variation. The authors concluded that HEX was not teratogenic at the levels tested (Murray et al., 1980).

Chernoff & Kavlock (1982) tested 28 compounds, including HEX, by an *in vivo* screening procedure. According to the researchers, the underlying hypothesis was that most prenatal insults would manifest themselves postnatally as reduced viability and/or impaired growth. Twenty-five Oravid CD-1 mice were administered HEX orally at or near the maternal minimal tolerated dose (MTD). The MTD was considered to be that dose resulting in either significant weight reduction during the treatment period, mortality, or other signs of toxicity. There were no differences in maternal weight gain, number of live offspring or average weight between the HEX-treated animals and controls when HEX was administered orally for 8-12 days at 45 mg/kg.

Gray & Kavlock (1984) extended the observation period proposed by Chernoff & Kavlock (1982, 1983) to 250 days to determine whether neonatal weight reductions persisted throughout life and whether other serious abnormalities or mortality resulted from exposure to HEX. CD-1 pregnant mice were orally exposed to HEX (45 mg/kg) on days 8 to 12 of gestation, which is within the period of major embryonic organogenesis. Females were weighed throughout dosing and on day 19 of gestation. They were allowed to deliver and the litters were counted and weighed at 1 and 3 days of age. The animals were observed at approximately 250 days of age. During the postmortem examination of males, body weight and the weights of the liver, testes, seminal vesicles, and right kidney were recorded. HEX did not produce any statistically significant developmental effects in this study.

Studies on the teratogenic potential of inhaled HEX were not found in the review of the scientific literature.

8.5 Mutagenicity

Goggelman et al. (1978) found that HEX was not mutagenic, either before or after liver microsomal activation, at 2.7 mmol/litre in an *Escherichia coli* K_{12} back-mutation system. In this test there was a 70% survival of bacteria at 72 h. HEX was not tested at higher concentrations because it was cytotoxic to *E. coli*. A previous report from the same laboratory (Greim et al., 1977) indicated that HEX was also non-mutagenic in *Salmonella typhimurium* strains TA1535 (base-pair mutant) and TA1538 (frame-shift mutant) after liver microsomal activation. However, no details of the concentrations tested were given. Although tetrachlorocyclopentadiene is mutagenic in these systems, probably through metabolic conversion to the dienone, it appears that the chlorine atoms at the C-1 position of HEX hinder metabolic oxidation to the corresponding acylating dienone (Greim et al., 1977).

A study conducted by the Industrial Bio-Test Laboratories (IBT, 1977) also suggested that HEX is not mutagenic in *S. typhimurium*. Both liquid HEX and its vapour were tested with and without metabolic activation. The vapour test was carried out in desiccators with the TA100 strain of *S. typhimurium* only. It is not clear from vapour test data that sufficient amounts of HEX or adequate exposure times (30, 60, and 120 min) were used. Longer exposures in the presence of HEX vapour may be necessary for a potential mutagenic effect to be seen.

At concentrations of up to 1.25 mg/litre in the presence of an S-9 liver activating system, HEX was not mutagenic in the mouse lymphoma mutation assay. Mutagenicity could not be evaluated at higher concentrations because of the cytotoxicity of HEX (Litton Bionetics, Inc., 1978a). This assay uses L5178Y cells that are heterozygous for thymidine kinase (TK+/-) and are sensitive. The mutation is scored by cloning with bromodeoxyuridine in the absence of thymidine. HEX is highly toxic to these cells, particularly in the absence of an activating system (at 0.04 ml/litre), and the positive control, dimethylnitrosamine, was mutagenic at 0.5 ml/litre.

Williams (1978) found that HEX (10^{-6} mol/litre) was inactive in the liver epithelial culture (hypoxanthine-guanine-phosphoribosyl transferase locus) mutation assay. At 10^{-5} mol/litre it also failed to stimulate DNA repair in hepatocyte primary cultures. Negative results were also obtained in an additional unscheduled DNA synthesis assay (Brat, 1983).

One study provided by the US National Toxicology Program (NTP) (Haworth et al., 1983) demonstrated a lack of mutagenicity of HEX (98% pure). In *S. typhimurium* strains TA98, TA100, TA1535, and TA1537, levels of up to 3.3 μg/plate were not mutagenic without activation, and levels of up to 100 μg/plate were not mutagenic after microsomal activation. Higher levels could not be tested because of excessive cell dealth. Zimmering et al. (1985) tested *Drosophila* by the sex-linked recessive lethal test (SLRL), either by feeding doses of 40 ppm for 3 days or by giving a single injection of 2000 ppm or 3000 ppm (volume not specified). The vehicle used was 10% ethyl alcohol, which did not totally dissolve the HEX. HEX (98%) was first assayed in the SLRL test in adult feeding experiments. When negative results were obtained, the chemical was retested by injecting < 1 day-old Canton-S wild-type *Drosphila* males. The results of the injection test were reported to be inconclusive.

HEX has also been assayed in the mouse dominant lethal test (Litton Bionetics, Inc., 1978b). In this assay, 0.1, 0.3, or 1.0 mg HEX/kg was administered by gavage to 10 male CD-1 mice for 5 days and the mice were then mated throughout spermatogenesis (7 weeks). This test determines whether the compound induces lethal genetic damage to the germ cells of males. There was no evidence of dominant lethal activity, at any dose level, based on any parameter (e.g., fertility index, implantations per pregnancy, average resorptions per pregnancy).

8.6 Cell transformation

The ability of HEX to induce morphological transformation of BALB/3T3 cells *in vitro* has been studied by Litton Bionetics, Inc. (1977).

The selection of test doses was based on previous cytotoxicity tests using a wide range of HEX concentrations at 0.0, 0.01, 0.02, 0.039, 0.078, and 0.156 mg per litre. The cultures were exposed for 48 h, which was followed by an incubation period of 3-4 weeks. The cultures were observed daily. The doses selected allowed a cell survival of 80-100% compared with controls (solvent only). This high survival rate permitted an evaluation of *in vitro* malignant transformation in cultures treated with HEX as compared with the solvent controls. 3-Methylcholanthrene at a dose level of 3 mg/litre was used as a positive control. Results indicated that HEX was not responsible for cell transformation.

8.7 Carcinogenicity

Bioassays of HEX for possible carcinogenicity have not been conducted. As noted previously (section 8.3.2), the NTP has completed a study on HEX for carcinogenicity by the inhalation route in rats and mice, but the results were not available when this monograph was being prepared.

9. EFFECTS ON HUMANS

9.1 General population exposure

There is very little detailed information available on the human health effects of HEX exposure. Acute human exposure has been reported in homes near waste sites where disposal of HEX has occurred (C.S. Clark et al., 1982; Elia et al., 1983). The odour threshold has been stated to be 1.92 $\mu g/m^3$ (0.17 ppb), but there appears to be great individual variation. According to a study completed by the A.D. Little Co. for the Occidental Chemical Corporation, the 100% panel recognition concentration was 1.92 $\mu g/m^3$ (0.17 ppb v/v)[a], but the study design and methodology were not reported. The US EPA (1982) estimated that exposure of the general population to HEX in air and/or water would be extremely low.

Treon et al. (1955) reported that members of a research group conducting toxicity tests developed headaches when they were accidentally exposed to unknown concentrations of HEX. The HEX escaped into the room when an aerated exposure chamber was opened.

In a 48-block area surrounding a contaminated sewer line in Kentucky, USA, questionnaires were sent to a selected sample of residents. A total of 212 occupants were surveyed. Only 3.8% of the residents reported an unusual odour. The most common symptoms were stomach aches (5.2%), burning or watery eyes (4.7%), and headaches (4.7%). There was no association between the frequency of symptoms and the distance of houses from the contaminated sewer line. No significant ambient air concentrations of HEX were found in these areas (Kominsky et al., 1978).

9.2 Occupational exposure

The US National Institute for Occupational Safety and Health (NIOSH, 1980) stated that 1427 workers were occupationally exposed to HEX. Officials from the Velsicol Chemical Corporation estimated that 157 employees had been

---

[a] Memorandum from G. Leonardos to P. Levins on Hooker special priority samples (odour properties).

potentially exposed to HEX in their production and processing facilities.

A well-documented incident of acute human exposure to HEX occurred in March 1977 at the Morris Forman Wastewater Treatment Plant in Louisville, Kentucky, USA (Wilson et al., 1978; Morse et al., 1979; Kominsky et al., 1980). The details of the incident are included in the original NIOSH Hazard Evaluation and Technical Assistance Report Number TA-77-39 (Kominsky et al., 1978), which is available from the US National Technical Information Service (NTIS). This treatment facility was contaminated with approximately 6 tonnes of HEX and octachlorocyclopentene, a waste product of HEX manufacture (Morse et al., 1979). The contamination was traced to an illegal dumping in one large sewer line that passed through several populated areas. Concentrations of HEX detected in the sewage at the plant were as high as 1000 mg/litre, and levels in the sewer line were up to 100 mg/litre. Air samples taken from the sewer line showed HEX concentrations to be as high as 4.5 mg/m^3 (400 ppb). Although the airborne concentrations of HEX at the time of the exposure in the treatment facility were not known, airborne concentrations in the primary treatment areas (screen and grit chambers) ranged between 3.05 and 10.96 mg/m^3 (270 and 970 ppb) 4 days after the plant had closed. It should be noted that the ACGIH 8 h-TWA for HEX was 0.1 mg/m^3 (10 ppb) in 1977. Workers tried to remove an odoriferous and sticky substance from the bar screens and grit collection system by using steam during clean-up of the contamination. This procedure produced a blue haze which permeated the primary treatment area. The airborne HEX concentration of the blue haze was reported to be 217 µg/m^3 (19.2 ppm) (Kominsky et al., 1980).

The US Centers for Disease Control (CDC) and NIOSH sent representatives to the plant with questionnaires about the type and duration of symptoms (Morse et al., 1979; Kominsky et al., 1980). In all, 193 employees were identified as having been potentially exposed for 2 or more days during the 2 weeks before the plant was closed (Morse et al., 1979). The questionnaire was sent to each of these 193 workers and 145 (75%) responded. Workers with complaints of mucous membrane irritation were given a physical examination, and blood and urine samples were collected for clinical screening by an independent laboratory. Data were also collected on the exposure levels and symptoms experienced by several people who had been acutely exposed to the chemical vapours.

The results of the CDC and NIOSH questionnaires showed that the odour of HEX had been detected by 94% of the workers before the onset of symptoms. The most common symptoms reported were eye irritation (59%), headaches (45%), and throat irritation (27%) (Table 18). Of the 41 plant workers examined, six had physical signs of eye irritation (i.e. lacrimation or redness) and five had signs of skin irritation. Laboratory analyses of blood and urine specimens from these workers showed marginal increases in lactic dehydrogenase activity in 27% of cases and proteinuria in 15%. Three weeks later, no abnormalities were detected in the blood and urine tests. After six weeks, some of the clinical symptoms persisted in 25-45% of the employees (Morse et al., 1978).

Table 18. Symptoms of 145 waste-water treatment plant employees exposed to HEX (Louisville, Kentucky, USA, March 1977)[a]

Symptom	No. of employees with symptoms	Percent of employees with symptoms
Eye irritation	86	59
Headache	65	45
Throat irritation	39	27
Nausea	31	21
Skin irritation	29	20
Cough	28	19
Chest pain	28	19
Difficult breathing	23	16
Nervousness	21	14
Abdominal cramps	17	12
Decreased appetite	13	9
Decreased memory	6	4
Increased saliva	6	4

[a] From: Morse et al. (1978).

Although there was difficulty in measuring the level of exposure received by the plant workers, more than 50%

of the clean-up crew were monitored. Laboratory tests showed no significant abnormalities in renal function tests, complete blood counts, or urinalysis, but several minimal or mild abnormalities were found in liver function tests (Kominsky et al., 1980). The abnormalities in 18 out of 97 clean-up workers are listed in Table 19. These people also had physical signs of mucous membrane irritation. A more detailed correlation between acute exposure level data and symptomatology was reported for nine adults (Kominsky et al., 1980). The data appear in Table 20. The exposure levels could not be estimated accurately because of prior exposure or because the worker had used protective equipment.

Table 19. Abnormalities detected in clean-up workers at the Morris Forman treatment plant, Louisville, Kentucky, USA[a]

Laboratory test	Normal range	Abnormal results	
		Range	No.[b]
Serum glutamate oxaloacetate transaminase	7-40 mU/ml	40-49	5
		50-59	1
		60-69	4
		70-79	0
		80-89	1
		90-99	1
Serum alkaline phosphatase	30-100 mU/ml	100-109	3
		110-119	1
		120-129	1
Serum total bilirubin	0.15-10 mg/dl	1.0-1.9	1[c]
Serum lactate dehydrogenase	100-225 mU/ml	230-239	1

[a] From: Kominsky et al. (1980).
[b] For individuals with more than one serial blood test, only the most abnormal result is tabulated.
[c] Associated with a serum glutamate oxaloacetate transaminase activity of 66 mU/ml.

Hazards to workers in treatment plants can result from chemical compounds contained in the industrial waste treated in municipal waste-water plants. The HEX-containing wastes from a pesticide manufacturer were treated in a municipal waste-water treatment plant at Memphis, Tennessee, USA. In 1978, the workers at this plant

Table 20. Individual exposure symptomatology correlations at the Morris Forman treatment plant (Louisville, Kentucky, USA)[a]

No. of workers	Estimated airborne exposure[b]	Immediate symptoms	Persistence of symptoms	Laboratory results
1	19.2 ppm HEX and 650 ppb OCCP for several seconds (no protective equipment)	lacrimation; skin irritation on face and neck; dyspnoea and chest discomfort; nausea (several min later)	1.5 h post-exposure: fatigue; erythema of exposed skin; eye irritation subsided in 1 day; chest discomfort persisted several days.	normal results 4 days post-exposure[c]
3	7083 ppb HEX and 446 ppb OCCP for several seconds. (half-face respirator)	lacrimation; irritation of exposed skin	asymptomatic at 2 h, except for for soreness around eyes	normal results 7 days post-exposure in one worker[c]
2	40-52 ppb HEX and 9-21 ppb OCCP (half-face respirator)	slight eye irritation	no symptoms after cessation of exposure	normal results 7 days post-exposure in one worker[c]
2	exact exposure unknown (half-face respirator)	slight skin irritation	faces felt "puffy" and "windburned" for 1-2 days after exposure; this was noted also by friends and family; no residual skin lesions.	none available
1	980 ppb HEX for 15 min; OCCP not measured (no protective equipment)	irritated eyes; nasal irritation and sinus congestion after 2 weeks of intermittent exposures	eyes felt "dry and irritated" for 2-3 days after exposure; nasal irritation ceased within 1-2 days of cessation of exposure.	none available

[a] From: Kominsky et al. (1980).
[b] OCCP = Octachlorocyc-opentene.
[c] Laboratory work was same as carried out on clean-up crew.

reported symptoms similar to those reported by workers in the Louisville plant referred to above. The air and wastewater were monitored, and analyses of urine and blood, liver function tests, and illness symptom questionnaires were completed. Workers from another waste treatment plant, where no pesticide wastes had been received, were used as a control group. No statistical differences in urine HEX concentrations or liver function tests between the exposed and control groups were found, although differences in levels of HEX-related compounds (co-contaminants) were detected (Elia et al., 1983).

9.3 Epidemiological studies

Mortality studies have been carried out on workers involved in the production of HEX or formulation of HEX products. Shindell et al. (1980) studied a cohort of 783 current and former workers who had been employed at the Velsicol Chemical Corporation plant at Marshall, Illinois, between 1946 and 1979. The purpose of the study was to evaluate the overall health status of all employees who had been present during the manufacture of chlordane for 3 months or more. There were no significant differences in mortality rates between these employees and the overall USA population. The observed value for deaths from all causes, including heart disease and cancer, was less than the expected value in the overall USA population.

Shindell et al. (1981) completed another epidemiological study for the Velsicol Chemical Corporation at its Memphis, Tennessee, plant covering the period 1952-1979. This coincided with the manufacture of heptachlor, a pesticide made from HEX. The reseachers studied 1115 current and former employees who had worked for 3 months or more. Again, there was no significant difference in mortality between the control and exposure groups.

Concomitant with the study performed by Shindell et al. (1980), Wang & MacMahon (1979) conducted a retrospective mortality study of workers employed at the Marshall and Memphis plants, where chlordane and heptachlor were manufactured between 1946 and 1976. They studied 1403 males who had worked at the plants for more than 3 months. There were 113 observed deaths compared with 157 expected deaths, giving a standardized mortality ratio (SMR) of 72.

Among the various causes of death, the two highest SMRs were 134 for lung cancer and 183 for cerebrovascular disease, but only the latter figure was statistically significant (P < 0.05). The excess mortality due to cerebrovascular disease was not related to the duration of exposure or to the latency period, and occurred only after termination of employment. Shindell & Ulrich (1986) updated their 1980 data set with additional worker data. There was no information specific to HEX exposure.

Buncher et al. (1980) studied the mortality of workers at a chemical plant that produced HEX. They examined 341 workers (287 male and 54 female), together with their health records, who had worked at the plant for at least 90 days between 1 October 1953 and 31 December 1974. Their vital status was determined through 1978. The expected numbers of deaths, based on the USA population and specific for sex, age, and calendar year, were calculated. The SMR for all causes of death was 69. Deaths caused by specific cancers, all cancers, and diseases of the circulatory and digestive systems were also fewer than expected. The authors noted that the time that had elapsed since the initial exposure (25 years at most) reduced the power of the study to detect cancers that may have a 10-40 year latent period.

Similar studies have been performed on a cohort of workers in the Shell International Petroleum plants in the Netherlands. These reports have been reviewed extensively in Environmental Health Criteria 91: Aldrin and Dieldrin (WHO, 1989).

10. EVALUATION OF HUMAN HEALTH RISKS AND EFFECTS ON THE ENVIRONMENT

10.1 Evaluation of human health risks

The general population is not at risk from exposure to HEX. However, people living near HEX processing and production facilities, as well as handlers of the chemical and its waste, are at risk. Exposure to HEX can occur through several different routes. However, HEX is much more toxic when inhaled than when ingested or following dermal contact. Skin exposure studies have shown that HEX can cause irritation, together with visceral changes that are similar to those that result from oral administration. Inhalation studies in animals have shown that HEX vapour is very irritating, repeated exposure to 1.13-2.26 mg/m^3 (0.1-0.2 ppm) causing pulmonary pathological changes. Acute toxic symptoms, including headaches, nausea, dizziness, and respiratory distress, have been reported. Based on a 90-day inhalation study in mice and rats, a NOEL of 0.45 mg/m^3 (0.04 ppm) has been estimated. No information is available on the long-term effects of a single exposure or of continuous exposure to HEX.

A carcinogenic study of HEX has been completed (but not evaluated) by the US National Toxicology Program. *In vitro* mutagenicity and cell transformation tests yielded negative results, as did an *in vivo* mouse dominant lethal assay at the levels tested. There was no evidence of teratogenicity in oral exposure studies in which three species were examined.

The toxic effects of HEX exposure on the human respiratory system are of major concern. Although the long-term toxicity data are limited, systemic toxic effects of HEX inhalation have been observed after short-term exposure, suggesting that long-term inhalation exposure to low concentrations of HEX could cause adverse health effects. Limited epidemiological studies of workers exposed to HEX at levels above those known to induce adverse health effects have been conducted, although concomitant exposure to other chemicals was known to have occurred. These workers complained of headaches, eye and skin irritation, nausea, dizziness, and respiratory distress, as did individuals living near areas where there were HEX releases.

10.2 Evaluation of effects on the environment

Release of HEX into the environment can result from the production, processing and use of HEX, disposal of waste containing HEX or from products contaminated with HEX. Only a small proportion of the total amount of HEX released into the environment from production, processing, and use can be expected to persist beyond a few days. However, waste disposal has resulted in HEX persisting in soil, sediment, and ground water. There is little monitoring information on the levels of HEX in air, water, and sediment. The exposure of organisms in the aquatic environment to HEX is therefore difficult to quantify.

HEX may undergo photolysis, hydrolysis, and biodegradation. In water, photolysis is the dominant process in direct sunlight, hydrolysis being the next most important degradation route. Volatilization to the atmosphere occurs from both water and soil. Biodegradation occurs in soil under both aerobic and anaerobic conditions and in sewage sludge. In water and aquatic sediment, biodegradation is initially limited. Information on the adaptation of microorganisms to degrade HEX is limited. HEX has a calculated tropospheric residence time of approximately 5 h.

Laboratory studies suggest that HEX is relatively immobile in soil, particularly in soil with a high organic content. However, leaching and movement in ground water has been reported in field studies.

HEX has been shown to be toxic to aquatic life at a level of 1-100 µg/litre. However, little information has been obtained under field conditions (long-term exposure at low concentration in the presence of sediment). The actual hazard to aquatic life is, therefore, difficult to assess. HEX is toxic to aquatic microorganisms but less toxic to soil microorganisms. Exposure of terrestrial organisms, except at or near disposal sites, would be expected to be low.

11. CONCLUSIONS AND RECOMMENDATIONS FOR PROTECTION OF HUMAN HEALTH AND THE ENVIRONMENT

11.1 Conclusions

- The general population is not at risk from exposure to HEX, except in the case of people residing near contaminated areas.

- The long-term human health effects of continuous low-level exposure are not known. Handlers of the product and its waste, as well as sewage workers, are at risk.

- Results of laboratory studies indicate that HEX should be degraded rapidly in the environment by photolysis, hydrolysis, or biodegradation. The relative importance of these processes varies with the medium. HEX is not a widespread environmental contaminant and the available data suggest that it is only found associated with production, processing and disposal sites. HEX does not bioaccumulate.

- Acute laboratory tests show that HEX is highly toxic to aquatic microorganisms, invertebrates, and fish, but less toxic to soil microorganisms. However, information obtained under environmentally realistic conditions is limited. The potential hazard to the general environment is expected to be low.

11.2 Recommendations for protection of human health and the environment

- Occupational exposure to HEX should be minimized by the use of closed systems. Guidelines for the disposal of HEX and HEX wastes should be followed.

- Environmental monitoring is needed to examine the persistence and fate of HEX in all media near production, processing and disposal sites, and also hazardous waste incinerators. Monitoring data are required for HEX in drinking-water, and in surface, shower, and ground water.

12. FURTHER RESEARCH

- Biomarker technology should be developed to indicate the possibility of past or current actions of HEX. Such biomarkers could be stable metabolites derived from HEX and its impurities that are present in the original preparation.
- Research is needed on the metabolic, degradative, and reactive products to understand the fate of HEX in human beings and the environment.
- Further study of the apparent disparity between degradation under laboratory conditions and that observed in the environment is needed.
- The efficacy and safety of current disposal methods should be evaluated and their present and future health impacts assessed.
- Developmental and reproductive studies of HEX need to be conducted, with emphasis on the inhalation route of exposure.
- Methods for the early warning of the presence of low levels of HEX should be developed.

REFERENCES

ABDO, K.M., MONTGOMERY, C.A., KLUWE, W.M., FARNELL, D.R., & PREJEAN, J.D. (1984) Toxicity of hexachlorocyclopentadiene: subchronic (13-week) administration by gavage to F344 rats and B6C3F$_1$ mice. J. appl. Toxicol., 4(2): 75-81.

ALEXANDER, D.J., CLARK, G.C., JACKSON, G.C., HARDY, C.J., STREET, A.E., HEYWOOD, R.H., BUIST, D., PRENTICE, D.E., & ISAACS, K.R. (1980) Subchronic inhalation toxicity of hexachlorocyclopentadiene in monkeys and rats, Huntingdon, Huntingdon Research Centre, 373 pp (Report VCL14M/791081) (Prepared for Velsicol Chemical Corporation, Chicago).

ATALLAH, Y.H., WHITACRE, D.M., & BUTZ, R.G. (1980) Fate of hexachlorocyclopentadiene in the environment. Paper presented at the 2nd Chemical Congress of the North American Continent, Las Vegas, Nevada, 29 August, 1980, Chicago, Velsicol Chemical Corporation.

BELL, M.A., EWING, R.A., & LUTZ, G.A. (1978) Reviews of the environmental effects of pollutants. XII. Hexachlorocyclopentadiene, Washington, DC, US Environmental Protection Agency (Report EPA-600/1-78-047) (NTIS PB 80-122963).

BENNETT, B. (1982) Hexachlorocyclopentadiene analyses of Mississippi river fish, Athens, Georgia, US Environmental Protection Agency, Region IV (Unpublished report).

BENOIT, F.M. & WILLIAMS, D.T. (1981) Determination of hexachlorocyclopentadiene at the nanogram per liter level in drinking water. Bull. environ. Contam. Toxicol., 27: 303-308.

BOYD, K.W., EMORY, M.B., & DILLON, H.K. (1981) Development of personal sampling and analytical methods for organochlorine compounds. In: Chemical hazards in the workplace, Washington, DC, American Chemical Society, pp. 49-64 (ACS Symposium Series No. 149).

BRAT, S.V. (1983) The hepatocyte primary culture/DNA repair assay on compound hexachlorocyclopentadiene using rat hepatocytes in culture, Valhalla, New York, American Health Foundation, Naylor Dana Institute for Disease Prevention.

BRIGGS, G.G. (1973) A simple relationship between soil adsorption of organic chemicals and their octanol/water partition coefficients. In: Proceedings of the 7th British Insecticide and Fungicide Conference, Brighton, England, 19-22 November, 1973, Croydon, British Crop Protection Council, Vol. 1, pp. 83-86 (Research Report).

BUA (BERATERGREMIUM FUR UMWELTRELEVANTE ALTSTOFFE) (1988) [Hexachlorocyclopentadiene] Weinheim, Germany, VCH Verlagsgesellschaft (BUA Report No. 25) (in German).

References

BUCCAFUSCO, R.J. & LEBLANC, G.A. (1977) Acute toxicity of hexachlorocyclopentadiene to bluegill (*Lepomis macrochirus*), channel catfish (*Ictalurus punctatus*), fathead minnow (*Pimephales promelas*), and the water flea (*Daphnia magna*) (Unpublished report prepared for Velsicol Chemical Corporation, Chicago).

BUNCHER, C.R., MOOMAW, C., & SIRKOSKI, E. (1980) Mortality study of Montague Plant-Hooker Chemical, Cincinnati, Ohio, University of Cincinnati Medical Center, Division of Epidemiology and Biostatistics (Unpublished report prepared for Hooker Chemical Corporation).

BUTZ, R.G. & ATALLAH, Y.H. (1980) Effects of hexachlorocyclopentadiene on three microbial functions (VCC Project No. 482428, Report No. 8) (Unpublished report prepared for Velsicol Chemical Corporation, Chicago).

BUTZ, R.G., YU, C.C., & ATALLAH, Y.H. (1982) Photolysis of hexachlorocyclopentadiene in water. Ecotoxicol. environ. Saf., 6: 347-357.

CALLAHAN, M.A., SLIMAK, M.W., GABEL, N.W., MAY, I.P., FOWLER, C.F., FREED, J.R., JENNINGS, P., DURFEE, R.L., WHITMORE, F.C., MAESTRI, B., MABEY, W.R., HOLT, B.R., & GOULD, C. (1979) Water-related environmental fate of 129 priority pollutants: II. Halogenated aliphatic hydrocarbons, halogenated ethers, monocyclic aromatics, phthalate esters, polycyclic aromatic hydrocarbons, nitrosamines, miscellaneous compounds, Washington, DC, US Environmental Protection Agency, Monitoring and Data Supervision Division, Office of Water Planning and Standards (Report EPA-440/4-79-029b).

CARTER, M.R. (1977) Legal affidavit field in the State of Georgia, Fulton County, dated 14 June, 1977. Testimony concerning estimates of total daily discharge of HEX from Velsicol Chemical Corporation, Atlanta, Athens, Georgia, US Environmental Protection Agency.

CHERNOFF, N. & KAVLOCK, R.J. (1982) An *in vivo* teratology screen utilizing pregnant mice. J. Toxicol. environ. Health, 10: 541-550.

CHERNOFF N. & KAVLOCK, R.J. (1983) A teratology test system which utilizes postnatal growth and viability in the mouse. In: Waters, M., Sandhu, S., Lewtas, J., Claxton, L., Chernoff, N., & Nesnow, S., ed. Short-term bioassays in the analysis of complex mixtures III, New York, London, Plenum Publishing Corporation, pp. 417-427.

CHOPRA, N.M., CAMPBELL, B.S., & HURLEY, J.C. (1978) Systematic studies on the breakdown of endosulfan in tobacco smokes: Isolation and identification of the degradation products from the pyrolysis of endosulfan I in a nitrogen atmosphere. J. agric. food Chem., 26: 255-258.

CHOU, S.F.J. & GRIFFIN, R.A. (1983) Soil, clay, and caustic soda effects on solubility, sorption and mobility of hexachlorocyclopentadiene, Springfield, Virginia, National Technical Information Service, 54 pp (PB 84-116060) (Environmental Geology Notes No. 104).

CHOU, S.F.J., GRIFFIN, R.A., CHOU, M.M, & LARSON, R.A. (1987)

Products of hexachlorocyclopentadiene (C-56) in aqueous solution. Environ. Toxicol. Chem., 6: 371-376.

CLARK, C.S., MEYER, C.R., GARTSIDE, P.S., MAJETI, V.A., & SPECKER, B. (1982) An environmental health survey of drinking water contamination by leachate from a pesticide waste dump in Hardeman County, TN. Arch. environ. Health, 37(1): 9-18.

CLARK, D.G., BLAIR, D., MARTIN, J., HENDY, R., PILCHER, A., & WIGGINS, D. (1982) Thirty-week chronic inhalation study of hexachlorocyclopentadiene (HEX) in rats, Tunstall, United Kingdom, Shell Toxicology Laboratory (Experiment No. 1760, Report No. SBGR.81) (Permission for use granted by M.J. Sloan, Shell Oil Co., Washington).

COLE, E.J. (1953) Chemotherapeutic and pharmacologic aspects of hexachlorocyclopentadiene, Laramie, University of Wyoming, Department of Veterinary Sciences and Bacteriology (Master's Thesis).

COLE, E.J. (1954) Treatment of sewage with hexachlorocyclopentadiene. Appl. Microbiol., 2: 198-199.

CUPITT, L.T. (1980) Fate of toxic and hazardous materials in the air environment, Research Triangle Park, North Carolina, US Environmental Protection Agency (Report EPA-600/3-80-084).

DAL MONTE, R.P. & YU, C.C. (1977) Water solubility of MC-984 and hex (Unpublished report prepared for Velsicol Chemical Corporation, Chicago).

DELEON, I.R., MABERRY, M.A., OVERTON, E.B., RASCHKE, P.C., REMELE, P.C., STEELE, C.F., WARREN, V.L., & LASETER, J.L. (1980a) Rapid gas chromatographic method for the determination of volatile and semivolatile organochlorine compounds in soil and chemical waste disposal site samples. J. chromatogr. Sci., 18: 85-88.

DELEON, I.R., BROWN, N.J., COCCHIARA, J.P., MILES, S.K., & LASETER, J.L. (1980b) Determination of trace levels of hexachlorocyclopentadiene and octachlorocyclopentene in body fluids. J. anal. Toxicol., 4: 314-317.

DILLON, H.K. (1980) Development of air sampling and analytical methods for toxic chlorinated organic compounds, Birmingham, Alabama, Southern Research Institute, 76 pp (NTIS PB 80-193279).

DOROUGH, H.W. (1979) The accumulation, distribution and dissipation of hexachlorocyclopentadiene (C56) in tissues of rats and mice, 27 pp (Unpublished report prepared for Velsicol Chemical Corporation, Chicago).

DOROUGH, H.W. (1980) Disposition of ^{14}C-hexachlorocyclopentadiene (C56) in rats following inhalation exposure, 53 pp (Unpublished report prepared for Velsicol Chemical Corporation, Chicago).

DOROUGH, H.W. & RANIERI, T.A. (1984) Distribution and elimination of hexachlorocyclopentadiene in rats and mice. Drug chem. Toxicol., 7(1): 73-89.

References

EICHLER, D.L. (1978) Quantitative analyses of mixtures containing trace amounts of pesticides. Internal memorandum to M.R. Zavon, Hooker Chemicals and Plastics Corporation, Niagara Falls, New York, 3 pp.

EL DAREER, S.M., NOKER, P.E., TILLERY, K.F., & HILL, D.L. (1983) Investigations on the basis for the differential toxicity of hexachlorocyclopentadiene administered to rats by various routes. J. Toxicol. environ. Health, 12: 203-211.

ELIA, V.J., CLARK, C.S., MAJETI, V.A., GARTSIDE, P.S., MACDONALD, T., RICHDALE, N., MEYER, C.R., VAN MEER, G.L., & HUNNINEN, K. (1983) Chemical exposure at a municipal wastewater treatment plant. Environ. Res., 32: 360-371.

EVANS, M.J., CABRAL-ANDERSON, L.J., & FREEMAN, G. (1978) Role of the Clara cell in renewal of the bronchiolar epithelium. Lab. Invest., 38: 648-655.

GOGGELMAN, W., BONSE, G., HENSCHLER, D., & CREIM, H. (1978) Mutagenicity of chlorinated cyclopentadiene due to metabolic activation. Biochem. Pharmacol., 27: 2927-2929.

GRAY, L.E., Jr & KAVLOCK, R.J. (1984) An extended evaluation of an *in vivo* teratology screen utilizing postnatal growth and viability in the mouse. Teratog. Carcinog. Mutagen., 4: 403-426.

GREIM, J., BIMBOES, D., GOGGELMANN, W., & KRAMER, M. (1977) Mutagenicity and chromosomal aberrations as an analytical tool for *in vitro* detection of mammalian enzyme-mediated formation reactive metabolites. Arch. Toxicol., 39: 159-169.

HAWLEY, G.G., ed. (1977) Condensed chemical dictionary, 9th ed., New York, Van Nostrand Reinhold Co.

HAWORTH, S., LOWLOR, T., MORTELMANS, K., SPECK, W., & ZEIGER, E. (1983) Salmonella mutagenicity test results for 250 chemicals. Environ. Mutagen., 5(Suppl. 1): 3-142.

HENDERSON, C. (1956) Bio-assay investigations for International Joint Commission, Niagara Falls, New York, Hooker Electrochemical Company, 17 pp (Unpublished report).

HUNT, G.E. & BROOKS, G.W. (1984) Source assessment for hexachlorocyclopentadiene, Research Triangle Park, North Carolina, Radian Corporation (Unpublished report prepared for the US Environmental Protection Agency).

IBT (1977) Mutagenicity of PCL-HEX incorporated in the test medium tested against five strains of *S. typhimurium* and as a volatilate against tester strain TA-100, Northbrood, Illinois, Industrial Bio-Test Laboratories.

IRDC (1968) Hexachlorocyclopentadiene and octachlorocyclopentene: Acute oral toxicity LD_{50} in male albino rats, Mattawan, Michigan, International Research and Development Corporation, 4 pp (Unpublished report prepared for Velsicol Chemical Corporation, Chicago).

IRDC (1972) Acute toxicity studies in rats and rabbits, Mattawan, Michigan, International Research and Development Corporation, 21 pp (Unpublished report prepared for Velsicol Chemical Corporation, Chicago).

IRDC (1978) Hexachlorocyclopentadiene: Teratology study in rats, Mattawan, Michigan, International Research and Development Corporation, 17 pp (Unpublished report prepared for Velsicol Chemical Corporation, Chicago).

IRISH, D.D. (1963) Halogenated hydrocarbons: II. Cyclic. Hexachlorocyclopentadiene. In: Patty, F.A., ed. Industrial hygiene and toxicology, 2nd revised ed., New York, Chichester, Brisbane, Toronto, John Wiley & Sons, pp. 1333-1363.

IRPTC (1989) IRPTC legal file, Geneva, International Register of Potentially Toxic Chemicals, United Nations Environment Programme.

KENAGA, E.E. (1980) Predicted bioconcentration factors and soil sorption coefficients of pesticides and other chemicals. Ecotoxicol. environ. Safety, 4: 26-38.

KENAGA, E.E. & GORING, C.A.I. (1980) Relationship between water solubility, soil sorption, octanol/water partitioning, and bioconcentration of chemicals in biota. In: Eaton, J.C., Parrish, P.R., & Hendricks, A.C., ed. Aquatic toxicology, Philadelphia, American Society of Testing and Materials, pp. 78-115 (ASTM STP 707).

KHAN, M.A.Q., SUDERSHAN, P., FEROZ, M., & PODOWSKI, A.A. (1981) Biotransformations of cyclodienes and their photoisomers and hexachlorocyclopentadiene in mammals and fish. In: Khan, M.A.Q. & Stanton, R.H., ed. Toxicology of halogenated hydrocarbons: Health and ecological effects, Oxford, New York, Pergamon Press, pp. 271-288.

KILZER, L., SCHEUNERT, I., GEYER, H., KLEIN, W., & KORTE, F. (1979) Laboratory screening of the volatilization rates of organic chemicals from water and soil. Chemosphere, 8: 751-761.

KLOSKOWSKI, R., SCHEUNERT, I., KLEIN, W., & KORTE, F. (1981) Laboratory screening of distribution, conversion and mineralization of chemicals in the soil-plant-system and comparison to outdoor experimental data. Chemosphere, 10: 1089-1100.

KOMINSKY, J.R. & WISSEMAN, C.L. (1978) Morris Forman wastewater treatment plant, Metropolitan Sewer District, Louisville, KY, Cincinnati, Ohio, National Institute of Occupational Safety and Health (NIOSH Hazard Evaluation and Technical Assistance Report No. TA 77-39) (NTIS PB 82-178088).

KOMINSKY, J.R., WISSEMAN, C.L., & MORSE, D.L. (1980) Hexachlorocyclopentadiene contamination of a municipal wastewater treatment plant. Am. Ind. Hyg. Assoc. J., 41: 52.

References

KOMMINENI, C. (1978) Pathology reports. Animal portion of the Louisville sewage study, Cincinnati, Ohio, National Institute of Occupational Safety and Health (NIOSH Report No. TA 77-39).

LAWLESS, E.W., VON RUMKER, R., & FERGUSON, T.L. (1972) The pollution potential in pesticide manufacturing, Springfield, Virginia, US Department of Commerce, National Technical Information Service (NTIS PB 213782/3) (Prepared for the US Environmental Protection Agency by Midwest Research Institute).

LAWRENCE, L.J. & DOROUGH, H.W. (1981) Retention and fate of inhaled hexachlorocyclopentadiene in the rat. Bull. environ. Contam. Toxicol., 26: 663-668.

LAWRENCE, L.J. & DOROUGH, H.W. (1982) Fate of inhaled hexachlorocyclopentadiene in albino rats and comparison to the oral and iv routes of administration. Fundam. appl. Toxicol., 2: 235-240.

LEVIN, A.A. (1982a) Hexachlorocyclopentadiene: Response to issues raised at US EPA Test Rules Meeting of March 17, 1982, Washington, DC, US Environmental Protection Agency, Office of Toxic Substances (Docket No. 40-8249078).

LEVIN, A.A. (1982b) Hexachloropentadiene: Follow-up and additional information to the 17 March, 1982 Meeting, Washington, DC, US Environmental Protection Agency, Office of Toxic Substances.

LICHTENBERG, J.J., LONGBOTTON, J.E., & BELLAR, T.A. (1987) Analytical methods for the determination of volatile non-polar organic chemicals in water and water-related environments. In: Suffet, I.H. & Malaiyandi, M., ed. Organic pollutants in water: Sampling, analysis and toxicity testing. A Symposium of the 188th Meeting of the American Chemical Society, Philadelphia, 29-31 August, 1984, Washington, DC, American Chemical Society, pp. 63-81.

LITTON BIONETICS, INC. (1977) Evaluation of hexachlorocyclopentadiene; *in vitro* malignant transformation in BALB/3T3 cells, Kensington, Maryland, Litton Bionetics, Inc., 7 pp (LBI Project No. 29840) (Prepared for Velsicol Chemical Corporation, Chicago).

LITTON BIONETICS, INC. (1978a) Mutagenicity evaluation of hexachlorocyclopentadiene in the mouse lymphoma forward mutation assay, Kensington, Maryland, Litton Bionetics, inc., 10 pp (LBI Project No. 20839) (Prepared for Velsicol Chemical Corporation, Chicago).

LITTON BIONETICS, INC. (1978b) Mutagenicity evaluation of hexachlorocyclopentadiene in the mouse dominant lethal assay, Kensington, Maryland, Litton Bionetics, Inc., 13 pp (LBI Project No. 20862).

LOOK, M. (1974) Hexachlorocyclopentadiene adducts of aromatic compounds and their reaction products. Aldrichem. Acta, 7(2): 1974.

LU, P.Y., METCALF, R.L., HIRWE, A.S., & WILLIAMS, J.W. (1975) Evaluation of environmental distribution and fate of hexachlorocyclopentadiene, chlordane, heptachlor, and heptachlor epoxide in a laboratory model ecosystem. J. agric. food Chem., 23: 967-973.

MACEK, R.J., PETROCELLI, S.R., & SLEIGHT, B.H., III (1979) Considerations in assessing the potential for, and significance of, biomagnification of chemical residues in aquatic food chains. In: Marking, L. & Kimerle, R.A., ed. Aquatic toxicology, Philadelphia, American Society for Testing and Materials, pp. 251-268.

MAYER, F.L. (1987) Acute toxicity handbook of chemicals to estuarine organisms, Gulf Breeze, Florida, US Environmental Protection Agency (Report EPA-600/8-017).

MEHENDALE, H.M. (1977) Chemical reactivity-absorption, retention, metabolism and elimination of hexachlorocyclopentadiene. Environ. Health Perspect., 21: 275-278.

MEIER, J.R., RINGHAND, H.P., COLEMAN, W.E., MUNCH, J.W., STREICHER, R.P., KAYLOR, W.H., & SCHENCK, K.M. (1985) Identification of mutagenic compounds formed during chlorination of humic acid. Mutat. Res., 157: 111-122.

MOLOTSKY, H.M. & BALLWEBER, E.G. (1957) Hexachlorocyclopentenones: US Patent No. 2,795,608, June 11, 1957, Chicago, Velsicol Chemical Corporation.

MORSE, D.L., LANDRIGAN, P.J., & FLYNT, J.W. (1978) Internal CDC report concerning hexachlorocyclopentadiene contamination of a municipal sewage treatment plant, Louisville, Kentucky, Atlanta, Georgia, Centers for Disease Control.

MORSE, D.L., KOMINSKY, J.R., & WISSEMAN, C.L., III (1979) Occupational exposure to hexachlorocyclopentadiene (How safe is sewage?). J. Am. Med. Soc., 241: 2177-2179.

MURRAY, F.J., SCHWETZ, B.A., BALMER, M.F., & STAPLES, R.E. (1980) Teratogenic potential of hexachlorocyclopentadiene in mice and rabbits. Toxicol. appl. Pharmacol., 53: 497-500.

NAS (1978) Kepone/mirex/hexachlorocyclopentadiene: An environmental assessment, Washington, DC, National Academy of Sciences (NTIS PB 280-289).

NEUMEISTER, C. & KURIMO, R. (1978) Determination of hexachlorocyclopentadiene and octachlorocyclopentene in air. Presented at the ACGIH Conference, Los Angeles, May 1978, Cincinnati, Ohio, American Conference of Governmental Industrial Hygienists.

NIOSH (1979) Manual of analytical methods, 2nd ed., Cincinnati, Ohio, National Institute for Occupational Safety and Health, Vol. 1-5 (DHEW (NIOSH) Pub. No. 77-157-A).

NIOSH (1980) Quarterly hazard summary report: Hexachlorocyclopentadiene, Cincinnati, Ohio, National Institute for Occupational Safety and Health.

NTP (1984a) Subchronic toxicity report on hexachlorocyclopentadiene (C53607) in B6C3F1 mice, Birmingham, Alabama, Southern Research Institute, 128 pp (Unpublished report prepared for the National Toxicology Program, National Institutes of Health, Birmingham, Alabama).

References

NTP (1984b) Subchronic toxicity report on hexachlorocyclopentadiene (C53607) in Fischer-344 rats, Birmingham, Alabama, Southern Research Institute, 196 pp (Unpublished report prepared for the National Toxicology Program, National Institutes of Health, Birmingham, Alabama).

OSHA (US DEPARTMENT OF LABOR, OCCUPATIONAL SAFETY AND HEALTH ADMINISTRATION) (1989) Air contaminants: Final rule - Hexachlorocyclopentadiene. Fed. Reg., 54(12): 2464.

PETERS, J.A., TACKETT, K.M., & EIMUTIS, E.C. (1981) Measurement of fugitive hydrocarbon emissions from a chemical waste disposal site. Presented at the 74th Annual Meeting of the Air Pollution Control Association, Philadelphia, 21-26 June, 1981, Dayton, Ohio, Montesanto Research Corporation.

PODOWSKI, A.A. & KHAN, M.A.Q. (1979) Fate of hexachlorocyclopentadiene in goldfish (Carassius auratus). Paper presented at the American Chemical Society Meeting, Honolulu, April 1979, Washington, DC, American Chemical Society.

PODOWSKI, A.A. & KHAN, M.A.Q. (1984) Fate of hexachlorocyclopentadiene in water and goldfish. Arch. environ. Contam. Toxicol., 13: 471-481.

RAND, G.M., NEES, P.O., CALO, C.J., ALEXANDER, D.J., & CLARK, G.C. (1982a) Effects of inhalation exposure to hexachlorocyclopentadiene on rats and monkeys. J. Toxicol. environ. Health, 9: 743-760.

RAND, G.M., NEES, P.O., CALO, C.J., CLARKE, G.C., & EDMONDSON, N.A. (1982b) The Clara cell: An electron microscopy examination of the terminal bronchioles of rats and monkeys following inhalation of hexachlorocyclopentadiene. J. Toxicol. environ. Health, 10: 59-72.

RIECK, C.E. (1977a) Effect of hexachlorocyclopentadiene on soil microbe populations, Lexington, Kentucky, University of Kentucky, Agronomy Department (Unpublished report prepared for Velsicol Chemical Corporation, Chicago).

RIECK, C.E. (1977b) Soil metabolism of ^{14}C-hexachlorocyclopentadiene, Lexington, Kentucky, University of Kentucky, Agronomy Department (Unpublished report prepared for Velsicol Chemical Corporation, Chicago).

RIECK, C.E. (1977c) Volatile products of ^{14}C-hexachlorocyclopentadiene, Lexington, Kentucky, University of Kentucky, Agronomy Department (Unpublished report prepared for Velsicol Chemical Corporation, Chicago).

ROBERTS, C.W. (1958) Chemistry of hexachlorocyclopentadiene. Chem. Ind., 1 February: 110.

SHELL RESEARCH LIMITED (1982) Toxicology of insecticide intermediates: The skin sensitizing potential of hexachlorocyclopentadiene, Tunstall, United Kingdom, Shell Research Ltd., Sittingbourne Research Centre (Report No. SBGR 82.225).

SHINDEL, S. & ULRICH, S. (1986) Mortality of workers employed in the manufacture of chlordane. An update. J. occup. Med., 28(7): 497-501.

SHINDELL & ASSOCIATES (1980) Report of epidemiologic study of the employees of Velsicol Chemical Corporation plant, Marshall, Illinois, January 1946-December 1979, Milwaukee, Wisconsin, Shindell and Associates (Unpublished report prepared for Velsicol Chemical Corporation, Chicago).

SHINDELL & ASSOCIATES (1981) Report of the epidemiologic study of the employees of Velsicol Chemical Corporation plant, Memphis, Tennessee, January 1952-December 1979, Milwaukee, Wisconsin, Shindell and Associates (Unpublished report prepared for Velsicol Chemical Corporation, Chicago).

SINHASENI, P., D'ALECY, L.G., HARTUNG, R., & SHLATER, M. (1982) Hexachlorocyclopentadiene increases oxygen consumption by intact rainbow trout and isolated heart mitochondria. Sixty-sixth Annual Meeting of the Federation of American Societies for Experimental Biology, New Orleans, 15-23 April, 1982. Fed. Proc., 41(5): 1580 (abstract).

SINHASENI, P., D'ALECY, L.G., HARTUNG, R., & SHLATER, M. (1983) Respiratory effects of hexachlorocyclopentadiene on intact rainbow trout (Salmo gairdneri) and on oxidative phosphorylation of isolated trout heart mitochondria. Toxicol. appl. Pharmacol., 67: 215-223.

SPEHAR, R.L., VEITH, G.D., DEFOE, D.L., & BERGSTEDT, B.A. (1977) A rapid assessment of the toxicity of three chlorinated cyclodiene insecticide intermediates to fathead minnows, Duluth, Minnesota, US Environmental Protection Agency, Environmental Research Laboratory (Report EPA-600/3-77-099).

SPEHAR, R.L., VEITH, G.D., DEFOE, D.L., & BERGSTEDT, B.A. (1979) Toxicity and bioaccumulation of hexachlorocyclopentadiene, hexachloronorbornadiene and heptachloronorbonene in larval and early juvenile fathead minnows, Pimephales promelas. Bull. environ. Contam. Toxicol., 21: 576-583.

SPRINKLE, C.L. (1978) Leachate migration from a pesticide. Waste disposal site in Hardeman County, Tennessee, Washington, DC, US Department of Interior, US Geological Survey (Waste Resources Investigations 78-128).

SRI (1980a) Acute toxicity report on hexachlorocyclopentadiene (C53607) in Fischer-344 rats and B6C3F1 mice, Birmingham, Alabama, Southern Research Institute, 44 pp (Unpublished report prepared for the National Toxicology Program).

SRI (1980b) Repeated-dose toxicity report on hexachlorocyclopentadiene (C53607) in Fischer-344 rats and $B6C3F_1$ mice, Birmingham, Alabama, Southern Research Institute, 33 pp (Unpublished report prepared for the National Toxicology Program).

SRI (1981a) Subchronic toxicity report on hexachlorocyclopentadiene (C53607) in $B6C3F_1$ mice, Birmingham, Alabama, Southern Research Institute, 137 pp (Unpublished report prepared for the National Toxicology Program).

SRI (1981b) Subchronic toxicity report on hexachlorocyclopentadiene (C53607) in Fischer-344 rats, Birmingham, Alabama, Southern Research Institute, 144 pp (Unpublished report prepared for the National Toxicology Program).

References

STEVENS, J.E. (1979) Chlorinated derivatives of cyclopentadiene. In: Kirk-Othmer encyclopedia of chemical technology, 3rd ed., New York, Chichester, Brisbane, Toronto, John Wiley & Sons, Vol. 5, pp. 791-797.

THIELEN, D.R., OLSEN, G., DAVIS, A., BAJOR, E., STEFANOVSKI, J., & CHODKOWSKI, J. (1987) An evaluation of microextraction/capillary column gas chromatography for monitoring industrial outfalls. J. chromatogr. Sci., 25(1): 12-16.

THUMA, N.K., O'NEILL, P.E., BROWNLEE, S.G., & VALENTINE, R.S. (1978) Biodegradation of spilled hazardous materials. In: Control of hazardous materials spills, Rockville, Maryland, Information Transfer, Inc., pp. 217-220.

TREON, J.F., CLEVELAND, F.P., & CAPPEL, J. (1955) The toxicity of hexachlorocyclopentadiene. Arch. ind. Health, 11: 459-472.

UNGNADE, H.E. & MCBEE, E.T. (1958) The chemistry of perchlorocyclopentenes and cyclopentadienes. Chem. Rev., 58: 249-254.

US EPA (1977) Chemical Hazard Information Profile: Hexachlorocyclopentadiene (CHIP), Washington, DC, US Environmental Protection Agency, TSCA Interagency Testing Committee.

US EPA (1980a) Summary of UWF Co-op Data on hexachlorocyclopentadiene and hexachlorobutadiene, Gulf Breeze, Florida, US Environmental Protection Agency, Environmental Research Laboratory (Unpublished laboratory data).

US EPA (1980b) Ambient water quality criteria for hexachlorocyclopentadiene, Washington, DC, US Environmental Protection Agency, Office of Water Planning and Standards (Report EPA-440/5-80-055) (NTIS PB 292-436).

US EPA (1980c) Ambient water quality criteria for hexachlorocyclopentadiene, Washington, DC, US Environmental Protection Agency, office of Water Regulations and Standards (Report EPA-440/5-80-055) (Unpublished data).

US EPA (1982) Hexachlorocyclopentadiene: Response to the Interagency Testing Committee. Fed. Reg., 47(250): 58023-58025.

US EPA (1989) Toxic chemical release inventory: Online printout of April 1989, Washington, DC, US Environmental Protection Agency (Available from the US National Library of Medicine).

VEITH, G.D., DEFOE, D.L., & BERGSTEDT, B.V. (1979) Measuring and estimating the bioconcentration factor of chemicals in fish. J. Fish. Res. Board Can., 36: 1040-1048.

VELSICOL CHEMICAL CORPORATION (1978) TSCA Sec. 8(E): Submission 8EHQ-06780208. Chlorinates in Mississippi River catfish and carp, 1978 (Unpublished report prepared for Velsicol Chemical Corporation, Chicago) (Submitted to the US Environmental Protection Agency, Office of Toxic Substances, Washington).

VELSICOL CHEMICAL CORPORATION (1979) Confirmation of HEX and HEX-BCH residues in human urine. Analytical method No. 0682, Chicago, Velsicol Chemical Corporation.

VELSICOL CHEMICAL CORPORATION (1984) Comments on draft health effects document for hexachlorocyclopentadiene, Chicago, Velsicol Chemical Corporation.

VELSICOL CHEMICAL CORPORATION (1986) Air sampling and monitoring at Velsicol production facilities, Chicago, Velsicol Chemical Corporation.

VERSCHUEREN, K. (1977) Handbook of environmental data on organic chemicals, New York, Van Nostrand Reinhold Co.

VILKAS, A.G. (1977) The acute toxicity of hexachlorocyclopentadiene to the water flea, *Daphnia magna straus*, Tarrytown, New York, Union Carbide Environmental Services (UCES Project No. 11506-03-05) (Prepared for Velsicol Chemical Corporation, Chicago).

WALSH, G.E. (1981) Effects of chlordane, heptachlor and hexachlorocyclopentadiene on growth of marine unicellular algae, Gulf Breeze, Florida, US Environmental Protection Agency, Environmental Research Laboratory (Unpublished report).

WALSH, G.E. (1983) Cell death and inhibition of population growth of marine unicellular algae by pesticides. Aquat. Toxicol., 3: 209-214.

WALSH, G.E. & ALEXANDER, S.V. (1980) A marine algal bioassay method: Results with pesticides and industrial wastes. Water Air Soil Pollut., 13: 45-55.

WANG, H.H. & MACMAHON, B. (1979) Mortality of workers employed in the manufacture of chlordane and heptachlor. J. occup. Med., 21: 745-748.

WEAST, R.C. & ASTLE, M.J. (1980) CRC handbook of chemistry and physics, 60th ed., Boca Raton, Florida, CRC Press, Inc.

WEBER, J.B. (1979) Adsorption of HEX by Cape Fear loam soil, Research Triangle Park, North Carolina State University (Unpublished report prepared for Velsicol Chemical Corporation, Chicago).

WHITMORE, F.C., DURFEE, R.L., & KHATTAK, M.N. (1977) Evaluation of a technique for sampling low concentrations of organic vapors in ambient air, Atlanta, Georgia, US Environmental Protection Agency (NTIS PB 279-672).

WHO (1989) Environmental Health Criteria 91: Aldrin and Dieldrin, Geneva, World Health Organization, 335 pp.

WILLIAMS, C.M. (1978) Liver cell culture systems for the study of hepatocarcinogens. Proceedings of the 12th International Cancer Congress, XII. International Cancer Congress Symposium No. 2: Chemical Oncogenesis and Mutagenesis, October 1978, New York, London, Plenum Publishing Corporation.

References

WILSON, J.A., BALDWIN, C.P., & MCBRIDE, T.J. (1978) Case history: Contamination of Louisville, Kentucky Morris Foreman treatment plant. Hexachlorocyclopentadiene. In: Control of hazardous material spills, Miami, Florida, Hazardous Material Control Research Institute, pp. 170-177.

WOLFE, N.L., ZEPP, R.G., SCHLOTZHAVER, P., & SINK, M. (1982) Transformation pathways of hexachlorocyclopentadiene in the aquatic environment. Chemosphere, 11(2): 91-101.

YOWELL, H.L. (1951) Fungicidal compositions containing hexachlorocyclopentadiene: US Patent 2538509, Washington, DC, US Patent Office.

YU, C.C. & ATALLAH, Y.H. (1977a) HEX hydrolysis at various pHs and temperatures, Chicago, Velsicol Chemical Corporation (Project No. 482428, Report No. 8) (Laboratory report).

YU, C.C. & ATALLAH, Y.H. (1977b) Photolysis of hexachlorocyclopentadiene, Chicago, Velsicol Chemical Corporation (Project No. 482428, Report No. 4) (Laboratory report).

YU, C.C. & ATALLAH, Y.H. (1981) Pharmacokinetics and metabolism of hexachlorocyclopentadiene in rats, Chicago, Velsicol Chemical Corporation (Project No. 482428, Report No. 10).

ZEPP, R.G., BAUGHMAN, G.L., & SCHLOTZHAUER, P.F. (1979) Dynamics of processes influencing the behavior of hexachlorocyclopentadiene in the aquatic environment. Paper presented at the 178th National Meeting of the American Chemical Society, Washington, 9-14 September, 1979, Washington, DC, American Chemical Society, Division of Environmental Chemistry.

ZIMMERING, S., MASON, J.M., VALENCIA, R., & WOODRUFF, R.C. (1985) Chemical mutagenesis testing in Drosophila. II. Results of 20 coded compounds tested for the National Toxicology Program. Environ. Mutagen., 7: 87-100.

APPENDIX 1

Information on guidelines, recommendations, and standards used in various countries is given in Table 21.

Table 21. Guidelines, recommendations and standards used in various countries/areas[a]

Country	Type	Medium/situation	Exposure limit description or remark	Value[b]	Date
Australia	recommendation	air/occupational	threshold limit value/time-weighted average short-term exposure limit	0.1 (0.01) 0.3 (0.03)	1983
Belgium	recommendation	air/occupational	threshold limit value/time-weighted average	0.1 (0.01)	1988
Canada	regulation	air/occupational	threshold limit value/time-weighted average	0.1 (0.01)	1980
Canada	regulation	transport	specific transportation regulations		1987
Finland	recommendation	air/occupational skin	time-weighted average short-term exposure limit	1.0 (0.1) 3 (0.3)	1989 1989
Netherlands	recommendation	air/occupational	time-weighted average/occupational	0.11 (0.01)	1986
Federal Republic of Germany	regulation	waste	"toxic waste" subject to specific handling, transport, treatment, storage, and disposal regulation/permits		1981
Switzerland	regulation	air/occupational	time-weighted average	0.1 (0.01)	1987
USA	regulation	water	ambient water quality criteria (organoleptic)	1 µg/litre	1980
USA (ACGIH)	recommendation	air/occupational	time-weighted average	0.1 (0.01)	1980

Table 21 (contd).

Country	Type	Medium	Description	Value	Year
USA	regulation	air/occupational	time-weighted average	0.1 (0.01)	1989
USA	regulation	water/land	notification of spill of 0.45 kg (1 lb) in 24-h period		1983
USA	regulation	waste transport	"toxic waste" subject to specific handling, transport, treatment, storage and disposal regulation/permits		1980
USA	draft recommendation	drinking-water	lifetime	7 µg/kg per day	1990
USSR	regulation	air/occupational	threshold limit value	0.01 (0.001)	1989
USSR	regulation	water	maximum allowable concentration	1 mg/litre	1985
USSR	regulation	air/ambient	short-term exposure limit	0.001	1987
Yugoslavia	regulation	air/occupational	time-weighted average	0.1	1985

[a] From: IRPTC (1989)
[b] Unless stated otherwise, units are mg/m^3. The value in parts per million is given in parentheses.

RESUME

L'hexachlorocyclopentadiène (HEX) est un liquide dense et ininflammable, de couleur jaune pâle à jaune verdâtre, et qui possède une odeur piquante caractéristique. Le HEX est très réactif; il donne lieu à des réactions d'addition et de substitution et à des réactions de Diels-Alder.

Aux Etats-Unis d'Amérique, la Velsicol Chemical Corporation est actuellement le seul producteur de HEX. En Europe, il est produit aux Pays-Bas par la Société Shell. Les chiffres de production sont confidentiels mais on estime que 3600 à 6800 tonnes de HEX sont produites actuellement aux Etats-Unis. En 1988, la production mondiale était d'environ 15 000 tonnes (BUA, 1988). Le HEX est utilisé comme intermédiaire dans la production de nombreux pesticides, mais quelques pays en ont limité l'emploi à la fabrication de certains pesticides organochlorés. Il est également utilisé pour la fabrication de retardateurs de flamme, de résines et de colorants.

Au cours de la production et de la transformation du HEX, de petites quantités sont libérées dans l'environnement. Ce peut être également le cas lorsqu'il constitue une impureté de certains des produits pour lesquels il sert d'intermédiaire. La libération de HEX peut intervenir pendant ou après le rejet. On ne dispose que de données limitées sur la surveillance des concentrations de cette substance dans l'environnement. D'après ces données, il semble que le HEX soit présent essentiellement dans le compartiment aquatique et y soit associé aux sédiments et aux matières organiques, sauf là où il y a eu rejet ou libération du produit. D'après les études en laboratoire, il y a sorption du HEX par la plupart des particules du sol. Toutefois, on a fait état d'un lessivage et d'un mouvement dans les eaux souterraines.

Aux Etats-Unis d'Amérique, on estime que 5,9 tonnes de HEX sont libérées annuellement dans le milieu (US EPA, 1989). En République fédérale d'Allemagne et aux Pays-Bas, environ 400 à 500 kg de HEX ont été libérés dans l'atmosphère en 1987 (BUA, 1988). En raison des propriétés physiques et chimiques du HEX, il ne devrait subsister qu'une faible fraction de ces émissions.

En s'appuyant sur les données de laboratoire disponibles, on a modélisé la destinée et le transport du HEX dans l'atmosphère et calculé que son temps de séjour dans la troposphère était d'environ 5 h. On a fait état d'un transport atmosphérique de HEX à partir d'une zone de stockage de déchets et de puits au cours du traitement de rejets industriels.

Dans l'eau, le HEX peut subir une photolyse, une hydrolyse et une biodégradation. Dans les eaux peu profondes son temps de demi-photolyse est inférieur à une heure. Dans les eaux plus profondes où la photolyse est exclue, le temps de demi-hydrolyse varie de plusieurs jours à environ trois mois et la biodégradation est encore beaucoup plus lente. Le HEX se volatilise à la surface de l'eau à une vitesse qui dépend de la turbulence et du degré de sorption par les sédiments.

En raison de sa faible solubilité dans l'eau, le HEX devrait être relativement immobile dans le sol. Toutefois on en a trouvé dans des eaux souterraines. La volatilisation de cette substance qui se produit très vraisemblablement à la surface du sol est d'autant plus importante que la teneur du sol en matières organiques est plus faible. Les résultats d'études en laboratoire indiquent que l'hydrolyse chimique et la métabolisation microbienne, qu'elles soient aérobie ou anaérobie, devraient réduire la teneur des sols en HEX.

En principe, le HEX devrait avoir un pouvoir de bioamplification notable en raison de sa forte lipophilicité (log du coefficient de partage octanol/eau). Toutefois les données expérimentales ne corroborent pas cette hypothèse. Des études sur animaux d'expérience ont montré que le ^{14}C-HEX est à la fois métabolisé et excrété dans les quelques heures qui suivent l'administration par voie orale, la rétention dans l'organisme étant très faible. Le facteur de bioconcentration à l'état stationnaire est inférieur à 30 chez les poissons. Les facteurs de bioaccumulation calculés à partir de modèles d'écosystèmes à court terme indiquent que le potentiel d'accumulation est modéré. Il semblerait donc que le HEX et ses métabolites ne persistent pas et ne s'accumulent pas en quantités importantes dans les systèmes biologiques.

On a montré qu'à faibles concentrations, le HEX était toxique pour la faune aquatique. Des cas de mortalité par

Résumé

intoxication aiguë (exposition de 48 à 96 h) ont été observés chez des crustacés et des poissons dulçaquicoles et marins à des concentrations nominales de 32 à 180 µg/litre, dans des systèmes statiques dont l'eau n'était pas renouvelée au cours de l'épreuve. Etant donné que le temps de demi-photolyse est inférieur à une heure, la concentration en HEX devrait avoir diminué de manière importante au cours de la période d'exposition utilisée dans ces études. Les seules études au cours desquelles on a mesuré les concentrations de HEX dans de l'eau courante ont donné une valeur de la CL_{50} à 96 h de 7 µg/litre pour le vairon américain et une crevette de mer. Les épreuves effectuées sur ces deux espèces ont donné, respectivement pour la CL_{10} et la CL_{40}, des valeurs de 3,7 et de 0,7 µg/litre.

Des épreuves statiques de sept jours effectuées sur des algues marines à des concentrations nominales allant de 3,5 à 100 µg/litre ont fait ressortir une réduction moyenne de la croissance (CE_{50}), qui était fonction de l'espèce. En milieu aqueux, le HEX est toxique pour de nombreux microorganismes à des concentrations nominales de 0,2 à 10 mg/litre, c'est-à-dire à des valeurs sensiblement plus importantes que celles qui sont nécessaires pour tuer la plupart des animaux et des plantes aquatiques. Le HEX semble être moins toxique pour les microorganismes terricoles que pour les microorganismes aquatiques, probablement en raison de l'adsorption du HEX sur la matrice constituée par le sol.

On pense que l'exposition devrait être faible mais les données actuellement disponibles sont insuffisantes pour permettre de déterminer les effets de l'exposition au HEX sur la flore et la faune terrestres.

La résorption du HEX non modifié est minimale du fait de sa réactivité vis-à-vis des membranes et des tissus de l'organisme et plus particulièrement, du contenu des voies digestives. Après administration par voie orale, percutanée ou par inhalation, la majeure partie du ^{14}C-HEX radiomarqué est retenue au niveau des reins, du foie, de la trachée et des poumons des animaux d'expérience. Une fois résorbé, le HEX est métabolisé et rapidement excrété, principalement dans les urines, un peu moins dans les matières fécales et à raison de moins de 1%, dans l'air expiré. La durée nécessaire pour l'élimination complète est d'environ 30 h quelle que soit la voie d'administration. Après inhalation ou administration par voie intraveineuse, le composé parent ne se retrouve plus dans les excréta; on a isolé des métabolites fécaux et urinaires mais ils n'ont pas été identifiés. C'est d'ailleurs la raison pour laquelle il est très difficile de se faire une idée de la pharmacocinétique du HEX et d'élucider son mode d'action.

La CL_{50} par inhalation (sur une période d'environ 4 h) est de 17,9 mg/m^3 chez le rat mâle et de 39,1 mg par m^3 chez la ratte. Bien qu'il existe quelques différences d'une espèce à l'autre, notamment entre les cobayes, les rats, les lapins et les souris, les vapeurs de HEX sont extrêmement toxiques pour toutes les espèces étudiées. C'est par inhalation qu'il se révèle le plus toxique, par comparaison avec l'administration orale ou percutanée, et il se montre également extrêmement irritant. Quelle que soit la voie d'administration, toute exposition aiguë entraîne des effets généraux pathologiques au niveau des poumons, du foie, des reins et des surrénales.

L'administration de HEX par voie orale à des rats (30 mg/kg et par jour) et à des souris (75 mg/kg et par jour) pendant 91 jours a déterminé une néphrose ainsi qu'une inflammation et une hyperplasie de l'estomac antérieur. On n'a pas relevé de signes manifestes après exposition de souris ou de rats à qui l'on avait fait inhaler du HEX à raison de 2,26 mg/m^3 (0,2 ppm), six heures par jour, cinq jours par semaine pendant 14 semaines. A la concentration de 1,69 mg/m^3 (0,15 ppm), on a observé seulement une petite irritation. Des rats exposés de la même manière à 5,65 mg/m^3 (0,5 ppm) de HEX pendant 30 semaines ont présenté des modifications histopathologiques au niveau du foie, des voies respiratoires et des reins. Une autre étude du même genre portant sur des rats et des souris et qui s'est prolongée pendant 90 jours a révélé des effets respiratoires à partir de 4,52 mg/m^3 (0,4 ppm). Le HEX ne s'est pas révélé mutagène lors d'épreuves *in vitro*, qu'il y ait ou non activation métabolique. Il s'est également révélé inactif dans les épreuves de dominance létale chez la souris. Administré par voie orale à des rats et à des

Résumé

souris, il ne s'est pas révélé tératogène, mais on ne dispose d'aucune donnée relative à sa tératogénicité éventuelle après exposition par voie respiratoire. On ne dispose que de données limitées sur l'exposition humaine au HEX et sur ses effets. On a observé des incidents isolés au cours desquels il y a eu forte irritation des yeux, du nez, de la gorge et des poumons. Cette irritation était généralement brève, les victimes commençant à récupérer dès cessation de l'exposition. Après une exposition de courte durée on n'a noté aucune différence statistiquement significative au niveau de certaines enzymes hépatiques entre les groupes exposés et les groupes témoins. On ignore quels peuvent être les effets à longue échéance sur la santé humaine d'une exposition continue à de faibles concentrations de HEX ou d'une exposition intermittente à des fortes concentrations. Les personnes qui sont amenées à manipuler cette substance ou des déchets qui en contiennent, ainsi que les égoutiers, travailleurs des usines de traitement d'eaux usées et personnes qui résident à proximité de décharges, pourraient être exposés au risque du fait des possibilités de contact avec cette substance ou avec les déchets qui résultent de sa fabrication.

La base de données dont on dispose n'est pas suffisante pour qu'on puisse évaluer la cancérogénicité du HEX. Le Programme toxicologique national des Etats-Unis (NTP) a procédé à des études d'inhalation sur des rats et des souris pendant toute la durée de leur vie. Une fois qu'un rapport sur la pathologie observée aura été publié, on aura une meilleure idée des effets à long terme éventuels de l'exposition au HEX. En ce qui concerne la cancérogénicité de cette substance, il faudra différer les travaux dans l'attente des résultats des épreuves effectuées par le NTP. Le Centre international de recherche sur le cancer a examiné les données existantes sur le HEX et l'a classé dans le Groupe 3 (ce qui indique qu'en raison d'insuffisances quantitatives ou qualitatives importantes, il n'est pas possible de déterminer, au vu des résultats disponibles, s'il y a présence ou absence d'effets cancérogènes). Un certain nombre d'études épidémiologiques sont citées dans la littérature; on n'a pas fait état d'une incidence accrue de cancers, de localisation quelconque, qui puisse être attribuée au HEX ou à ses métabolites.

RESUMEN

El hexaclorociclopentadieno (HEX) es un líquido denso de color amarillo pálido o verdoso, no inflamable, con un olor acre característico. Su masa molecular relativa es de 272,77 y es poco soluble en agua. El HEX es muy reactivo y experimenta reacciones de adición, sustitución y de Diels-Alder.

En los EE.UU., la Velsicol Chemical Corporation es la única empresa que actualmente produce HEX. En Europa lo fabrica la Shell Chemical Corporation en los Países Bajos. Los datos de producción son propiedad de las empresas, pero se calcula que al año se producen en los EE.UU. entre 3600 y 6800 toneladas de HEX. En 1988, la producción mundial fue de aproximadamente 15 000 toneladas (BUA, 1988). Aunque el HEX se utiliza como intermedio en la producción de numerosos plaguicidas, algunos países han restringido su empleo en la fabricación de ciertos plaguicidas organoclorados. También se utiliza en la producción de pirorretardantes, resinas y tintes.

Durante la fabricación y elaboración del HEX, se liberan pequeñas cantidades de la sustancia al medio ambiente. También puede liberarse cuando aparece en forma de impureza en algunos de los productos para los que sirve de intermedio. El HEX puede liberarse tanto durante como después de su evacuación. Sólo se dispone de datos limitados de vigilancia de los niveles ambientales de HEX. Esos datos indican que aparece principalmente en el compartimento acuático y que se asocia a los sedimentos y la materia orgánica del fondo salvo en los lugares en los que se ha producido evacuación o liberación. En el laboratorio, el HEX se adsorbe sin dificultad a la mayoría de los tipos de partículas del suelo. Sin embargo, se han comunicado casos de lixiviación y de movimiento en aguas subterráneas.

En los EE.UU., se calcula que la liberación total de HEX al medio ambiente en un año es de 5,9 toneladas (US EPA, 1989). En la República Federal de Alemania y los Países Bajos, se emitieron en 1987 alrededor de 400-500 kg (BUA, 1988). Dadas las características físicas y químicas del HEX, es de esperar que solo persista una pequeña fracción de esas emisiones.

Basandose en los datos de laboratorio disponibles, se ha formulado un modelo sobre el destino y el transporte del HEX en la atmósfera y se ha calculado que tiene un tiempo de residencia de aproximadamente 5 horas en la troposfera. Se ha comunicado la existencia de transporte atmosférico de HEX desde una zona en la que se almacenan desechos y a partir de las cisternas durante el tratamiento de desechos industriales.

En el agua, el HEX puede experimentar fotolisis, hidrólisis y biodegradación. En aguas poco profundas, tiene una semivida fotolítica de < 1 h. En aguas más profundas, donde la fotolisis se ve impedida, se ha observado que la semivida hidrolítica puede variar entre varios días y aproximadamente tres meses, mientras que es de prever que la biodegradación se produzca con más lentitud. Se sabe que el HEX se volatiliza en las aguas superficiales, y que la tasa de volatilización varia con la turbulencia y con la adsorción a los sedimentos.

Debido a su baja solubilidad en el agua, el HEX debe ser relativamente inmóvil en el suelo. Sin embargo, se ha detectado la sustancia en aguas subterráneas. La volatilización, que tiene más probabilidades de producirse en la superficie del suelo, guarda relación inversa con los niveles de materia orgánica en éste. Los resultados de estudios en laboratorio indican que la hidrólisis química y el metabolismo microbiano, tanto aeróbico como anaeróbico, deben reducir los niveles de HEX en los suelos.

En teoría, el potencial de biomagnificación del HEX debe ser importante debido a su elevada lipofilia (log coeficiente de partición octanol/agua). Este extremo, sin embargo, no ha sido demostrado en pruebas experimentales. Los estudios en animales de laboratorio han demostrado que el ^{14}C-HEX es metabolizado y excretado durante de las primeras horas que siguen la administración de una dosis por vía oral, y que la proporción que queda retenida en el organismo es pequeña. En los peces, los factores de bioconcentración en estado estable son < 30. Los factores de bioacumulación derivados de modelos de ecosistemas a corto plazo indican un moderado potencial de acumulación. Así pues, parece que el HEX y sus metabolitos no persisten ni se acumulan en gran medida en los sistemas biológicos.

Se ha demostrado que el HEX en bajas concentraciones es tóxico para los organismos acuáticos. Se ha observado

Resumen

letalidad en exposiciones agudas (48 a 96 h) en crustáceos y peces de agua dulce y salada, en concentraciones nominales de 32-180 µg/litro en sistemas de exposición estática en los que el agua no se renovó durante la prueba. Puesto que la semivida fotolítica es < 1 h, la concentración de HEX habría disminuido sustancialmente durante el periodo de exposición utilizado en esos estudios. En los únicos estudios en los que se usó agua corriente y se midieron las concentraciones de HEX, se obtuvieron valores de la CL_{50} en 96 horas de 7 µg por litro en *Pimephales promelas* y un camarón de mar. Los ensayos realizados con esas dos especies dieron un valor de CL_{10} de 3,7 y un valor de CL_{40} de 0,7 µg por litro, respectivamente.

En ensayos estáticos de siete días con algas marinas se observó una reducción mediana del crecimiento (CE_{50}) a concentraciones nominales que variaron entre 3,5 y 100 µg/litro, según la especie.

En medios acuosos, el HEX resulta tóxico para numerosos microorganismos en concentraciones nominales de 0,2-10 mg/litro, es decir, niveles sensiblemente mayores que los necesarios para destruir a la mayoría de los animales o vegetales acuáticos. El HEX parece menos tóxico para los microorganismos en el suelo que en el medio acuático, probablemente a causa de la adsorción del HEX a la matriz del suelo.

Aunque cabe esperar que la exposición sea reducida, actualmente no se dispone de bastante información para determinar los efectos de la exposición al HEX en la vegetación o la fauna terrestres.

La absorción de HEX sin modificar es mínima debido a su reactividad con las membranas y los tejidos del organismo y especialmente con el contenido del tracto gastrointestinal. La mayor parte del ^{14}C-HEX radiomarcado queda retenido en el riñón, el hígado, la tráquea y los pulmones de los animales tras la administración por vía oral, cutánea o respiratoria. El HEX absorbido es metabolizado y excretado rápidamente, sobre todo en la orina, menos en las heces y < 1% en el aire expirado. El tiempo de eliminación terminal es de unas 30 horas, con independencia de la vía de administración. Tras la inhalación o la administración intravenosa, no se excreta HEX sin modificar; los metabolitos fecales y urinarios se han aislado pero no se han identificado. La falta de identificación de los metabolitos representa uno de los principales obstaculos para evaluar la farmacocinética y los mecanismos potenciales de acción del HEX.

En la rata, la CL_{50} aguda por inhalación (durante un periodo de aproximadamente 4 h) es de 17,9 mg/m^3 en el macho y 39,1 mg/m^3 en la hembra. Aunque hay algunas diferencias interespecíficas entre cobayos, conejos, ratas y ratones, los vapores de HEX son sumamente tóxicos para todas las especies ensayadas. Su toxicidad parece máxima cuando se administra por inhalación, en comparación con la administración oral y cutánea, y es un irritante primario fuerte. Los efectos sistémicos de la exposición aguda, con independencia de la vía de administración, comprenden cambios patológicos en el pulmón, el hígado, el riñón y las glándulas suprarrenales.

La administración oral a corto plazo a ratas (38 mg/kg al día) y ratones (75 mg/kg al día) durante 91 días produjo nefrosis e inflamación e hiperplasia de la región anterior del estómago. No se observaron signos manifiestos cuando se expuso a ratas o ratones por inhalación a 2,26 mg/m^3 (0,2 ppm), 6 h/día, 5 días/semana, durante 14 semanas. Con 1,69 mg/m^3 (0,15 ppm) sólo se observó una ligera irritación. La exposición de ratas a la inhalación de 5,65 mg/m^3 (0,5 ppm) durante 30 semanas provocó cambios histopatológicos en el hígado, el tracto respiratorio y el riñón. En un estudio de inhalación a corto plazo de HEX en ratones y ratas durante 90 días se observaron efectos en el sistema respiratorio a 4,52 mg/m^3 (0,4 ppm) o más. No se ha demostrado que el HEX sea mutagénico en ensayos *in vitro,* con o sin activación metabólica. También resultó inactivo en ensayos de letalidad dominante en el ratón. Tampoco se ha demostrado que sea teratogénico en ratas y ratones por exposición oral; no se dispone de datos sobre la teratogenicidad del HEX tras la exposición por inhalación.

Sólo se dispone de datos limitados sobre los efectos de la exposición al HEX en la salud humana. Se han producido incidentes aislados en los que el HEX provocó fuerte irritación de los ojos, la nariz, la garganta y los pulmones. Por lo general esa irritación fue breve, y la

Resumen

recuperación se inició en cuanto cesó la exposición. No se observaron diferencias estadísticamente significativas en ciertas enzimas hepáticas entre grupos expuestos y grupos testigo tras la exposición a corto plazo. Se desconocen los efectos a largo plazo en la salud humana de la exposición continua a bajos niveles y/o la exposición aguda intermitente. Se ha demostrado que los manipuladores del producto y de sus desechos, así como las personas que trabajan en la depuración de aguas residuales o que viven en las proximidades de los lugares de evacuación corren riesgo debido al potencial de exposición a la sustancia química o a los residuos de su fabricación.

La base de datos no es lo bastante amplia ni adecuada para evaluar la carcinogenicidad del HEX. El Programa Nacional de Toxicología de los EE. UU. ha llevado a cabo un bioensayo de inhalación durante toda la vida en ratas y ratones. Cuando se publique el informe patológico, se comprenderá mejor los efectos a largo plazo de la exposición al HEX. La evaluación de la carcinogenicidad deberá demorarse hasta que estén disponibles los resultados del bioensayo del Programa. El Centro Internacional de Investigaciones sobre el Cáncer evaluó los datos existentes para el HEX y clasificó la sustancia en el Grupo 3 (lo que indica que, debido a limitaciones importantes de orden cualitativo o cuantitativo, no puede interpretarse que los estudios demuestren ni la existencia ni la ausencia de efecto carcinogénico). En la bibliografía se citaron varios estudios epidemiológicos; no se notificaron aumentos de la incidencia de neoplasmas en ninguna localización que pudieran atribuirse al HEX o sus metabolitos.